Contents

Aids to Anaesthesia
Clinical Practice

For Churchill Livingstone

Publisher: Michael Parkinson
Project Editor: Janice Urquhart
Copy Editor: Michael Fitch
Indexer: Nina Boyd
Design Direction: Erik Bigland
Project Controller: Frances Affleck

Aids to Anaesthesia Clinical Practice

T. E. J. Healy MSc MD MRCS FRCA
Emeritus Professor of Anaesthesia,
The University of Manchester, Manchester, UK

B. J. Pollard BPharm MD FRCA
Professor of Anaesthesia, The University of Manchester,
Manchester, UK

SECOND EDITION

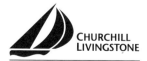

CHURCHILL
LIVINGSTONE

EDINBURGH LONDON NEW YORK PHILADELPHIA SYDNEY TORONTO 1999

CHURCHILL LIVINGSTONE
An imprint of Harcourt Brace and Company Limited

First published 1984
Second edition 1999

ISBN 0 443 04233 0

British Library Cataloguing in Publication Data
A catalogue record for this book is available from the British Library.

Library of Congress Cataloging in Publication Data
A catalog record for this book is available from the Library of
Congress.

The
publisher's
policy is to use
paper manufactured
from sustainable forests

Printed In China
EPC/01

Preface

This book is intended as an aid to candidates preparing for postgraduate examinations in the clinical practice of anaesthesia. The success of the first edition has indicated to us that a second edition is warranted. Many sections have been extensively rewritten to reflect changes in practice and to bring it fully up to date.

The application of physiological and pharmacological concepts to medical problems in clinical anaesthesia is dealt with on a functional basis. Where possible, the appropriate pathological process is identified and the measures intended to minimise the hazard due to the disturbance are presented. A more conventional approach is used in the description of techniques used in clinical practice.

The style is deliberately concise and aims to be a distillation of knowledge. It therefore complements the major textbooks and does not in any way seek to attempt to replace them. This book is essentially an aide-memoire.

The authors would like to express thanks to Mrs Caroline Madourie who uncomplainingly typed and edited the manuscripts.

B. J. P.
T. E. J. H.   Manchester 1998

1. Principles of general anaesthesia

The classic 'triad' of anaesthesia consists of hypnosis, analgesia and suppression of reflexes. This is often extended to include a fourth component of anaesthetic practice—the maintenance of gaseous exchange. A number of authorities replace suppression of reflexes with muscle relaxation. The original triad may therefore be expanded into five points. The roots of anaesthesia lie in a technique in which a single agent was administered in a relatively large dose to secure all the requirements of the anaesthetic. Modern anaesthesia commonly employs a number of drugs each with a single primary effect (e.g. hypnosis, analgesia or neuromuscular blockade), which are combined in low doses (balanced anaesthesia) to allow the minimum effective dose of each to be used.

INTRAVENOUS AGENTS

Hypnotic agents induce anaesthesia and usually have no analgesic action. Respiratory and cardiovascular depression may occur, particularly if used in association with other drugs which have a central depressant effect. A hangover effect may occur, as may tolerance, psychological dependence and enzyme induction if the agents are administered for a prolonged period of time. The last mentioned may lead to altered metabolism of other medication including oral anticoagulants, corticosteroids, digoxin, oestrogen and androgens.

INTRAVENOUS HYPNOTICS USED TO INDUCE GENERAL ANAESTHESIA

Barbiturates

Thiopentone and methohexitone are derivatives of barbituric acid (Fig. 1.1). Although basically lipophilic, they are made water-soluble by preparation of the sodium salt. Depression of synaptic transmission in the reticular activating system is thought to be the principal mechanism leading to sleep, although recent evidence has suggested that they may enhance chloride flux at GABA receptors. This mechanism is different from that of the benzodiazepines on the GABA system. Sensory pathways are not depressed and there is no analgesic effect—indeed the pain threshold may be reduced. The EEG initially shows increased activity with high-amplitude waves at a frequency of approximately

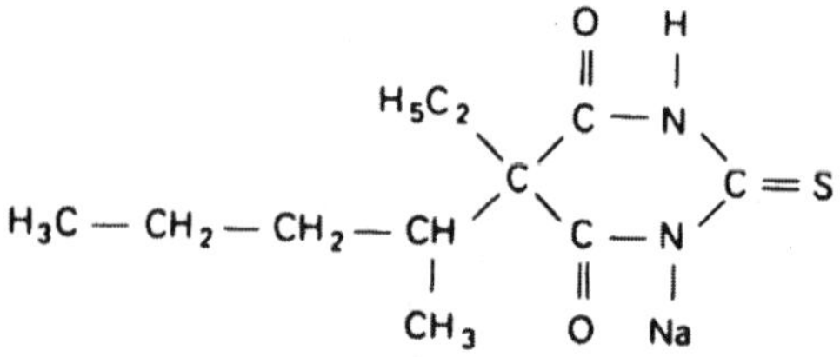

Thiopentone

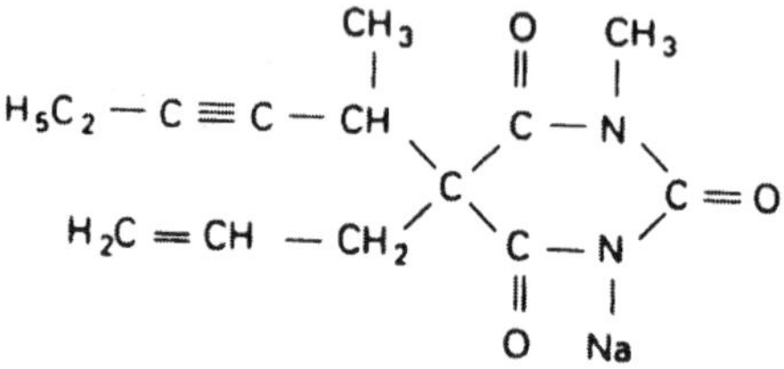

Methohexitone

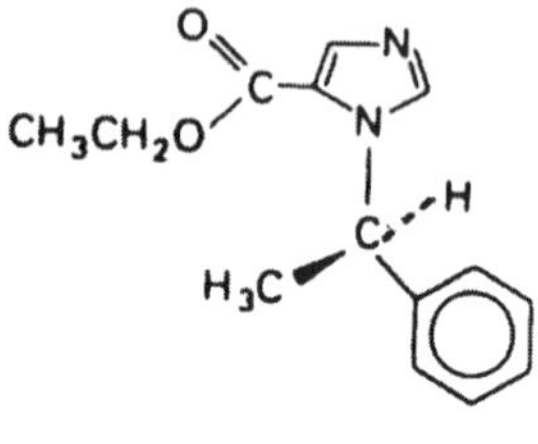

Etomidate

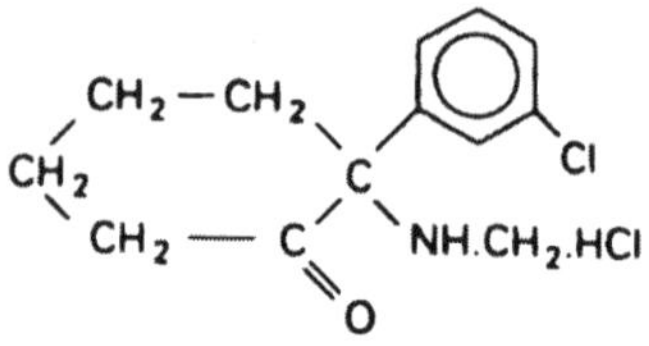

Ketamine

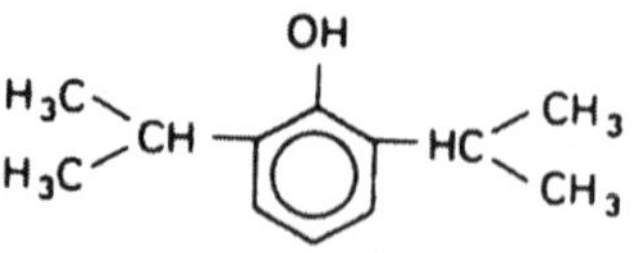

Propofol

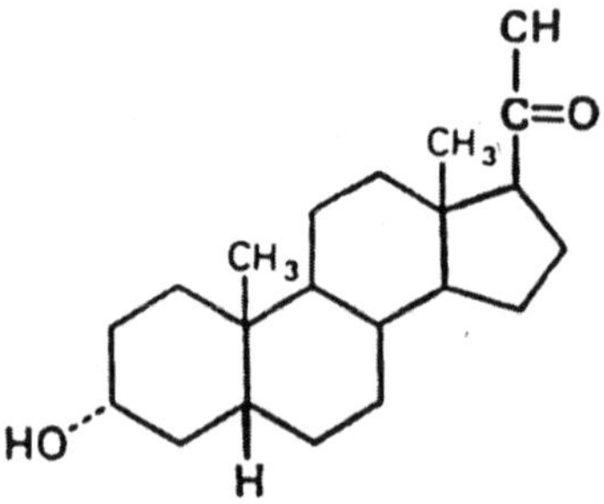

Eltanolone

Fig 1.1   Structural formulae of the common intravenous induction agents.

10–30 Hz, but with loss of consciousness slow waves (delta rhythm), similar to those seen in physiological sleep, occur.

Thiopentone and methohexitone have a high lipid–water solubility coefficient and therefore the onset of effect is rapid (10–20 s). They are subsequently redistributed to other tissues, e.g. muscle and fat, and therefore have a brief duration of action (about 5–10 min) in spite of a relatively slow metabolism (approximately 15% per hour for thiopentone). Methohexitone has a more rapid clearance (1–2 hours). These barbiturates are almost completely metabolised and excretion of metabolic products is increased in the presence of alkaline urine.

Thiopentone dissolves to form an alkaline solution (pH 11.6 for 2.5% solution) which is irritant to tissues—extravasation may lead to local tissue sloughing. Intra-arterial injection may cause intense vasoconstriction with thrombosis, leading to gangrene of the limb extremity (finger tips). Treatment includes direct intra-arterial injection of vasodilating agents such as procaine, papaverine or tolazoline and blockade of the sympathetic nerves (stellate ganglion block or axillary brachial plexus block). Methohexitone is less irritant than thiopentone but may be associated with laryngospasm, hiccup and abnormal muscle movements.

Benzodiazepines

Benzodiazepines have many actions in common, although the degree to which a particular action predominates varies from drug to drug. Intramuscular absorption is poor in spite of good oral absorption. Highly protein-bound, many of these drugs have a prolonged plasma half-life and are metabolised to active metabolites which also have a prolonged half-life.

Enterohepatic recirculation and hepatic storage may lead to reappearance of the effects of the drugs after apparent recovery. Their effects include anxiolysis, sedation, amnesia, muscular relaxation (centrally mediated), confusion, allergic phenomena and mild respiratory depression. They have anticonvulsant properties but no significant analgesic effect. Their action may be potentiated by other central depressants. Benzodiazepines are principally used as anxiolytics, premedicants, anticonvulsants, to control athetoid movements in spasticity, and for sedation for minor procedures. Variation in response to a given dose makes them unsatisfactory for use as induction agents. Their general safety has been greatly increased by the introduction of flumazenil, a specific benzodiazepine antagonist.

Propofol

Di-isopropyl phenol (Fig. 1.1) is not soluble in water and is presented in a lipid emulsion. Anaesthesia is induced in one arm–brain circulation time and a single bolus dose of 2–3 mg/kg will last for about 3–5 minutes. It is a negative inotrope and produces vasodilation resulting in occasional hypotension which is less marked if given slowly. It is not an analgesic but does suppress laryngeal reflexes and has antiemetic properties. The rapid recovery from propofol is due to redistribution. It is, however, rapidly metabolised in liver (beta half-life 50 min), so being suitable for total intravenous anaesthesia by infusion and also for day patients. Pain on injection is a problem particularly when it is injected into a small vein in the back of the hand—but this can be reduced by adding 20 mg lignocaine to the syringe before injection.

Phencyclidine derivatives

The only pheneyclidine derivation of relevance to anaesthesia is ketamine (Fig. 1.1). It may be administered i.v., i.m. or p.r. Unconsciousness follows within 30–40 s of i.v. injection (1–2 mg/kg) and lasts for 5–8 minutes. Onset is slower when it is given by other routes (5–10 mg/kg i.m. or p.r.). Ketamine produces a dissociative state characterised by catalepsy, sedation, amnesia and analgesia. The eyelash and laryngeal reflexes may not be lost and there may be an increase in muscle tone. Recovery follows redistribution with subsequent metabolism to active metabolites (elimination half-life is approximately 2–5 hours). During recovery, vivid dreaming and irrational behaviour may occur. The analgesic effect persists into the recovery period.

In spite of having, like other anaesthetic agents, a generalised depressant effect, a rise in heart rate, blood pressure and myocardial oxygen consumption usually follows an i.v. injection of ketamine. This sympathomimetic action is due partly to noradrenaline re-uptake blockade and partly to a central stimulant effect. It has a use in the management of bronchospasm, but should be avoided in hypertensive patients. Diplopia and nystagmus may also occur, as may tonic and clonic muscle movements. Despite these drawbacks, ketamine is useful for repeated minor procedures in children and also has a place in military applications.

Ketamine is a racemic mixture. Recent evidence has suggested that more of the unwanted effects may be associated with the R(–) isomer than the S(+) isomer, the latter being 3–4 times more potent than the former. The central action of ketamine is mediated, at least in part, through the NMDA receptor.

Steroids

Alphaxalone formulated with alphadalone for. i.v. injection was marketed as Althesin. Despite being a smooth and pleasant anaesthetic agent it was withdrawn because of a number of acute hypersensitivity reactions which lead to cardiovascular collapse and severe bronchospasm. These may have been caused by the cremophor vehicle rather than the steroid agent.

Another steroid derivative, 5-beta pregnanolone (Eltanolone, Fig. 1.1) has undergone clinical trials. It is insoluble in water and formulated as an emulsion. The induction dose is approximately

0.6 mg/kg and anaesthesia is induced in one arm–brain circulation time. Recovery is rapid with minimal hangover. There is a dose-related fall in blood pressure although respiratory depression appears to be less than with propofol. There is no pain on injection. It has a high therapeutic index but is not yet available for clinical use.

Carboxylated imidazole

Etomidate (Fig. 1.1) has a rapid onset of action after i.v. injection (induction dose 0.2–0.3 mg/kg) and rapid recovery. There is little change in the respiratory or cardiovascular systems and it is therefore a suitable induction agent for the high-risk patient. Etomidate may produce involuntary movement and local pain during intravenous injection. The incidence of postoperative nausea and vomiting is slightly greater than with the other i.v. induction agents. Etomidate suppresses adrenocortical function and is therefore not suitable for use by prolonged infusion.

ANALGESIA

Analgesics are drugs which relieve pain and fall into two broad categories:

- The antipyretic or anti-inflammatory analgesics, which are primarily used for pain of musculoskeletal origin and act through a peripheral mechanism
- Narcotic or opioid analgesics, which are primarily used for severe pain of visceral origin and for pre-, post and intra-operative pain. They act through a central mechanism.

NON-STEROIDAL ANTI-INFLAMMATORY DRUGS (NSAIDs)

The members of this heterogeneous group of compounds possess analgesic, anti-inflammatory and antipyretic properties to varying degrees. In the context of anaesthesia they are usually given for their analgesic action.

The original NSAID was acetylsalicylic acid (aspirin), an effective analgesic with antipyretic and anti-inflammatory actions. Plasma concentration rises rapidly following oral administration and maximum plasma concentration is achieved within 2–3 hours. Acetylsalicylic acid is hydrolysed in the gastric mucosa and plasma to form the salicylate. Approximately 60% of plasma salicylate is bound to protein and is rapidly distributed throughout the body. It is important to reduce the dose of other simultaneously used drugs which are also protein-bound, e.g. warfarin, as these may be displaced from their protein-binding sites by salicylate.

Salicylate increases the bleeding time by decreasing platelet adhesiveness and by reducing plasma prothrombin levels. Renal excretion of salicylate is encouraged by an alkaline urine, and conversely, in an acid urine, reduced ionisation of salicylate leads to reduced excretion.

Salicylate stimulates breathing by a direct central action and by increasing oxygen utilisation and carbon dioxide production. There is also uncoupling of phosphorylating mechanisms. In salicylate poisoning there may be a metabolic acidosis, a respiratory alkalosis and occasionally there may be a rise in P_aCO_2 with a fall in pH. Overdose may lead to headache, dizziness, tinnitus, thirst, nausea and skin eruptions.

Aspirin is not routinely used in anaesthesia due mainly to its unwanted side-effects. It is often administered in small doses in the management of transient cerebral ischaemic episodes and acute myocardial infarction. There are a number of newer NSAIDs which, although not devoid of side-effects, produce less problems than aspirin. These include ketorolac, diclofenac, ketoprofen, ibruprofen and piroxicam, several of which are available as parenteral preparations.

The NSAIDs all act by inhibition of cyclo-oxygenase (COX). This enzyme is known to exist in at least two forms and there are large differences in the spectrum of action of the various NSAIDs on COX subtypes. The therapeutic effect appears to relate to an action on COX subtype I whereas the principal side effects correlate with inhibition of COX subtype II. This may, in part, explain the differences in side-effect profiles of the newer agents. The effects on COX are all reversible except for aspirin which irreversibly inhibits COX.

OPIOID ANALGESICS

Morphine and drugs with similar action are sometimes described as 'narcotic analgesics' but should more correctly be described as 'opioids.' The effects and potencies of these drugs are commonly compared with morphine as the standard and their use may lead to physical dependence. Their action is mediated through central opioid receptors which exist widely distributed through the brain and spinal cord.

Naturally occurring alkaloids
Only three of the many alkaloids in the seed capsule of the opium poppy *Papaver somniferum* remain in clinical use. These are morphine, codeine and papaverine. The central effects of morphine include analgesia, euphoria and sedation. Depression of the cough reflex, respiratory centre and vasomotor centre also occur, together with nausea, vomiting and miosis. Oliguria is associated with the release of antidiuretic hormone. Peripheral effects include reduced gastrointestinal tone, constipation, spasm of the biliary tract and contraction of the sphincter of Oddi. Histamine release may lead to bronchospasm. Morphine is concentrated in the lungs, liver, kidney, spleen and skeletal muscle. Hepatic conjugation is followed by excretion primarily in the urine and to a lesser extent in bile.
A single dose of morphine is largely excreted within 24 h.
The 6-glucuronide metabolite is active and is more slowly excreted.

Codeine (methylmorphine) is less potent than morphine, its metabolic product. It has very little tendency to produce respiratory depression. It is used for cough suppression as well as analgesia. It may cause constipation and is used to treat diarrhoea. It is often used for analgesia in neurosurgical units.

Papaveretum contains a mixture of the water-soluble alkaloids of opium. The analgesic effect primarily depends on its morphine content which is standardised to 50% of the mixture. Its side-effects are as for morphine and it is regarded as being more sedative than morphine.

Diacetylmorphine (heroin) is a synthetic derivative of morphine. It is more lipid-soluble than morphine and better absorbed orally. It is a pro-drug, being converted to morphine in the tissues. It is more potent, more sedative and more addictive than morphine, but causes less respiratory depression and has a shorter duration of action.

Dihydrocodeine is more potent than codeine but has very little respiratory or cardiovascular depression. This drug is used as an oral analgesic for mild to moderate pain.

Synthetic opioids

Pethidine was the first wholly synthetic opioid. It has a shorter duration of action and is less potent than morphine but is less likely to produce spasm of smooth muscle. Nausea, vomiting and sedation occur and it may release histamine in higher doses. It must be avoided in patients taking monoamine oxidase inhibitors (MAOIs).

Fentanyl is a phenylpiperidine derivative which is approximately 80 times more potent than morphine. It is highly lipid-soluble and over 80% protein-bound. The peak effect of fentanyl is reached within 5 minutes of i.v. injection and although it has a fairly short clinical duration of action this is due to redistribution. It is metabolised in the liver to inactive products with an elimination half-life of about 4 hours, which explains its longer action duration in higher doses. Fentanyl is a potent respiratory depressant with little or no effect on the cardiovascular system. It is used extensively as an analgesic supplement to general anaesthesia.

Alfentanil is a fentanyl analogue with a potency of about one-tenth that of fentanyl. Its onset is more rapid and its duration of action shorter than that of fentanyl (due to redistribution). It is metabolised in the liver with an elimination half-life of under 2 hours. It has a similar respiratory depressant action and cardiovascular stability to fentanyl.

Sufentanil is another fentanyl analogue which is ten times more potent than fentanyl and produces more sedation than fentanyl. The onset is rapid and duration of action is similar to that of fentanyl but it has a shorter elimination half-life (2–3 hours). It shows the same effects, side effects and clinical applications as fentanyl. It is not currently available in the UK.

Remifentanil is the newest opioid and is characterised by a rapid onset and a very short duration of action. It is metabolised in the plasma by an esterase (not cholinesterase) with an elimination half-life of 10–20 min and therefore really requires to be administered by continuous infusion. Its analgesic potency, effects and side effects are essentially similar to those of fentanyl.

Pentazocine is an opioid analgesic with antagonistic properties and may therefore precipitate the withdrawal syndrome in opiate addicts. Dysphoria may follow its use. It may be administered intravenously, intramuscularly, subcutaneously or orally. Its popularity is waning.

Buprenorphine, a thebaine, derivative, is a very potent analgesic with partial agonist properties. In addition to analgesia, buprenorphine may produce sedation, respiratory depression and miosis although effective analgesia usually occurs in association with negligible respiratory depression. Dysphoria and hallucinatory effects have not been reported but nausea and vomiting may be troublesome in ambulant patients. It may be administered i.v., i.m., s.c. or sublingually. A single dose provides prolonged pain relief, thereby reducing the need for repeated doses. It undergoes high first-pass metabolism and so cannot be administered orally.

Tramadol acts at central opioid receptors and also at central serotonin and central adrenergic receptors. Its potency is similar to that of pethidine. It has a low addiction potential. The tendency to produce respiratory depression is less than that of other opioids but it possesses anticholinergic side effects, particulary dry mouth, dizziness, sedation and sweating.

Antiemetics

When an opioid analgesic is prescribed, an antiemetic should also be available. In those patients who are particularly susceptible to nausea and vomiting after surgery and anaesthesia the administration of an antiemetic with the pre-med or during the procedure is useful. Nausea and vomiting is one of the commonest reasons for delayed discharge home of the day patient and a prophylactic antiemetic is particularly useful in this patient population. The most effective antiemetics are the 5HT3 antagonists (e.g. ondansetron). Metoclopramide and prochlorperazine are also popular. A small dose of droperidol is a potent antiemetic but unpleasant subjective side effects occasionally occur in a minority of patients.

NEUROMUSCULAR BLOCKADE

The tone in a muscle is adjusted by proprioceptive responses and voluntary control. Muscular contraction is initiated centrally via alpha motor neurons and is under voluntary control. Muscle tissue is depressed by general anaesthetic agents and therefore deep anaesthesia is associated with a reduction in muscle tone and in the force of artificially induced contraction. Interference in the motor nerve pathway will reduce the muscle contraction response and also muscle tone. This is most commonly achieved by using a neuromuscular blocking agent. Muscular relaxation may also be produced by the use of centrally acting drugs such as benzodiazepine or baclofen although these drugs have no direct effect on the neuromuscular junction. Motor impulse transmission can also be interrupted in the nerve fibres within the vertebral canal by the use of local anaesthetic agents injected into either the subarachnoid or the epidural space. Neuromuscular transmission is mediated by a chemical transmitter (acetylcholine) released from the nerve ending. Acetylcholine is synthesised in the nerve ending where it is stored in vesicles. The arrival of an action potential down in the nerve triggers the release of acetylcholine which diffuses across to the motor end-plate on the muscle surface. The motor end-plate is a highly specialised area of the post-synaptic membrane. The attachment of acetylcholine to its receptors leads to a change in the membrane permeability to sodium and potassium ions and depolarisation occurs. The depolarisation process is then propagated across the muscle fibre and muscle contraction results. Acetylcholine is rapidly hydrolysed by acetylcholinesterase and repolarisation of the membrane takes place.

DEPOLARISING AGENTS

Depolarising agents produce initial depolarisation of the end-plate membrane and then prevent repolarisation, thereby maintaining blockade of neuromuscular transmission. Recovery follows drug removal from the neuromuscular junction.

Suxamethonium

Suxamethonium is the only depolarising relaxant presently available. Suxamethonium is injected as a 1–2 mg/kg bolus dose. Its effect is short-lived and a single bolus dose lasts about 4–6 minutes and is terminated following hydrolysis by plasma cholinesterase (pseudocholinesterase). The use of suxamethonium may be associated with severe postoperative muscle pains, the incidence of which may be reduced by the prior injection of a small dose of a non-depolarising agent.

The action of suxamethonium may be prolonged if cholinesterase activity is impaired. Reduced plasma cholinesterase levels are associated with severe liver disease, chronic anaemia, cardiac failure, bronchial neoplasia, starvation, exposure to organophosphorus compounds including ecothiopate iodide, radiotherapy and treatment with immunosuppressive or anti-neoplastic agents or an anticholinesterase, e.g. neostigmine.

A low level of plasma cholinesterase activity may be associated with congenital atypical cholinesterase. This condition occurs in about 1 in 3000 patients and is genetically determined by a pair of non-dominant allelomorphic autosomal genes. The various

possibilities produce a range of activities from zero to normal.
Patients can be screened by measurement of plasma cholinesterase
level. The original laboratory screening techniques used the
differences in inhibition of activity by dibucaine and fluoride. The
activity of the atypical enzyme is resistant to inhibition by dibucaine
(cinchocaine), fluoride or both whereas the activity of the normal
enzyme is inhibited by both dibucaine and fluoride. This fact provides
a basis for identifying the presence or absence of an atypical gene.

The administration of a dose of suxamethonium usually results
in a rise in serum potassium of between 0.5 and 1.0 mmol/l. Care
should therefore be taken in patients with an already elevated
potassium. There are a number of conditions in which suxamethonium
produces an exaggerated rise in potassium; these include burns,
demyelinating diseases and major nerve trunk lesions, including
spinal cord transection. It should be avoided in these patients.

Malignant hyperpyrexia and profound bradycardia in children may
follow the use of suxamethonium. Bradycardia is more common
following a second dose of suxamethonium, and a suitable vagolytic
agent (atropine or glycopyrrolate) should be administered.

NON-DEPOLARISING AGENTS

Non-depolarising relaxants bind to the postsynaptic membrane
but do not excite a change in membrane permeability, so that
depolarisation does not occur. The result is that access by
acetylcholine to the receptors is reduced. A dynamic equilibrium
exists between acetylcholine and the muscle-relaxant molecules
such that shortly after administration of the relaxant, drug molecules
bias the equilibrium in their favour, and block results. A subsequent
increase in the available acetylcholine following administration of
an anticholinesterase (e.g. neostigmine) alters the equilibrium and
the block is reduced. Effective drugs include d-tubocurarine,
pancuronium atracurium, vecuronium, rocuronium, mivacurium,
doxacurium, pipecuronium and cisatracurium (Table 1.1). The
neuromuscular blocking effect may be potentiated by other agents
which are anti-cholinergic (anti-nicotinic), which include drugs with
a ganglion-blocking action such as trimetaphan. Agents which
reduce acetylcholine release potentiate the non-depolarising
relaxants, and this includes the aminoglycoside antibiotics,
disopyramide, verapamil and nifedipine. The effect of muscle
relaxants may also be modified by lithium salts, the intravenous
injection of local anaesthetic agents, and by changes in plasma
electrolyte concentration.

Tubocurarine
This relaxant is little used now but is of historical interest, being
the original naturally occurring relaxant. Mild hypotension may
result from a combination of ganglion blockade and histamine
release. This drug should therefore be used with care when

Table 1.1 Pharmacodynamic and pharmacokinetic data for the non-depolarising muscle relaxants

	ED_{95} mg/kg	Onset (min)	Clinical duration (min)	Elimination half-life (min)	Spontaneous recovery index (min)
Tubocurarine	0.5	4–6	80–120	100–200	25–35
Pancuronium	0.06	4–6	80–120	90–120	25–30
Atracurium	0.23	3–5	30–40	20–22	10–15
Cistracurium	0.05	2–4	40–50	20–22	10–15
Vecuronium	0.05	3–5	30–40	60–120	10–15
Rocuronium	0.3	2–3	30–40	60–120	10–15
Mivacurium	0.08	3–5	20–25	5–9	6–10
Doxacurium	0.03	8–14	80–200	70–100	–
Pipecuronium	0.05	5–7	80–120	75–120	30–40

Note
These data are averages taken from multiple sources. Onset refers to a typical intubating dose and clinical duration is the duration of that dose up to recovery of the first twitch of a train of four to 25%. The spontaneous recovery index is the time taken to recover from 75% block to 25% block in the absence of an anticholinesterase.

combined with drugs which lower blood pressure, and caution must be exercised in the presence of phaeochromocytoma, a history of bronchial asthma or relative hypovolaemia. The effect is reduced by alkalosis and prolonged by acidosis. The ED_{95} is 0.5 mg/kg, onset 4–5 min and duration of action 45–60 min.

Pancuronium
This synthetic steroid-based agent has a slightly more rapid onset than tubocurarine (3–4 min) and an action duration of about 45–60 min. It does not lead to histamine release or hypotension. Tachycardia and a rise in blood pressure may occur, as a result of noradrenaline re-uptake blockade. The ED_{95} is 0.08 mg/kg. It is metabolised to 3-hydroxy (active), 17-hydroxy (inactive) and 3,17-dihydroxy (inactive) compounds which are excreted in the urine.

Atracurium
This highly selective intermediate acting non-depolarising muscle-relaxant is broken down by three pathways. It is degraded spontaneously by the non-enzyme decomposition process Hofmann elimination (approximately 40% in the normal individual), destroyed by an esterase in the liver (approximately 60%) and potentially (< 1%) by an esterase in the blood (not plasma cholinesterase). Its elimination kinetics are therefore independent of liver or kidney insufficiency. It has good cardiovascular stability but histamine release may result from larger bolus doses. Its ED_{95} is 0.23 mg/kg, onset 2–3 min and duration of action 20–30 min.

Vecuronium
This synthetic steroid-based agent is almost devoid of histamine-releasing potential. It possesses excellent cardiovascular stability. It is metabolised, like pancuronium, to the 3-hydroxy, 17-hydroxy and 3,17-dihydroxy compounds, the first of which has a potency about 70% of vecuronium itself. These are excreted in the urine and the duration of action of vecuronium may thus be prolonged in renal failure. The ED_{95} is 0.04 mg/kg, onset about 2–3 min and duration of action 20–30 min.

Rocuronium
Another steroid-based agent, rocuronium, is the fastest-onset non-depolarising agent presently available. It is associated with a slight tachycardia. No metabolites have so far been detected in man. It is eliminated in both bile and urine and its action is prolonged in the presence of liver failure. Its ED_{95} is 0.3 mg/kg, onset 1–2 min and duration of action 20–30 min.

Mivacurium
Structurally related to atracurium, mivacurium has the shortest duration of action (12–15 min) of the non-depolarising agents. It may produce histamine release and hypotension following a rapid bolus dose and has a relatively slow onset (3–5 min) in normal clinical doses. It is metabolised by plasma cholinesterase to inactive compounds and its duration of action is prolonged in patients with decreased plasma cholinesterase activity. The ED_{95} is 0.08 mg/kg.

Doxacurium
This long-acting agent is related to atracurium. It has impressive cardiovascular stability and is almost devoid of side-effects. It has an ED_{95} of 0.03 mg/kg, onset time of 4–7 min and duration of action of 60–75 min. It is presently only available in North America.

Pipecuronium
Originating from Eastern Europe, this relaxant has excellent cardiovascular stability. It is long-acting (60–75 min), has a relatively slow onset (3–6 min), and is rarely used in the U.K. The ED_{95} is 0.05 mg/kg.

Cisatracurium
This is one of the component isomers of atracurium. It possesses about 60% of its activity but only comprises 15% of the racemic mixture. It shares the same metabolic pathways as atracurium. Its cardiovascular stability is greater than that of atracurium and it has negligible histamine-releasing potential. Its ED_{95} is 0.05 mg/kg, onset 2–4 min and duration of action 40–50 min.

INHALATIONAL ANAESTHETIC AGENTS

Some inhalational agents at low concentration possess hypnotic properties but at higher concentrations produce analgesia and muscle relaxation. Others in low concentrations produce analgesia with very little sedation, e.g. trichloroethylene. Potency is expressed in terms of the MAC value, which is the minimum alveolar concentration of the agent, at equilibrium, required to prevent 50% of patients moving during a 'standard' skin incision at normal atmospheric pressure. The oil/gas partition coefficient bears a close relation to the MAC value (Table 1.2).

Nitrous oxide

A gas, neither flammable nor explosive, stored as a liquid under pressure at room temperature. The blood/gas solubility coefficient of 0.47 explains the rapid onset. Its potency is low, however, as reflected in the high MAC value (105%). A good analgesic at inspired concentrations of 50–70%, it has no effect on skeletal, cardiac or uterine muscle. During recovery, rapid nitrous oxide diffusion into the alveoli may reduce alveolar oxygen tension (P_aO_2) and lead to hypoxia (diffusion hypoxia—Fink effect).

Diethyl ether

A volatile liquid, boiling point 36.5°C, flammable in air or oxygen. Induction and recovery are slow (blood/gas solubility coefficient 12.1), but its potency is high (MAC 1.92%). Diethyl ether is irritant to the airway but nonetheless produces bronchodilatation. Raised sympathetic tone masks the depressant effect on the heart. Respiratory depression occurs at high concentrations. It is now rarely used but is nonetheless one of the safest volatile anaesthetic agents.

Table 1.2 Physicochemial properties of volatile anaesthetic agents

	MAC (%)	Oil/gas solubility coefficient	Blood/gas solubility coefficient	Boiling point (°C)	SVP (mmHg)
Nitrous oxide	105	1.4	0.47	– 89	*
Halothane	0.75	224	2.3	50.2	243
Enflurane	1.68	96	1.9	56.5	172
Isoflurane	1.13	91	1.4	48.5	240
Desflurane	6.1	19	0.42	23.5	664
Sevoflurane	2.1	53	0.60	58.5	160
Diethyl ether	1.92	65	12.1	36.5	425

Notes
SVP = saturated vapour pressure in mmHg at 20°C.
*Nitrous oxide is a gas at room temperature and its SVP is so high as to be meaningless.

Halothane
A volatile liquid with a boiling point of 50°C, neither flammable nor explosive. Induction and recovery are rapid (blood/gas solubility 2.3) and potency is high (MAC 0.75%). Tachypnoea may lead to reduced alveolar ventilation, and, as the inhaled concentration is increased, myocardial depression may result in hypotension. The fall in cardiac output is related to a reduced stroke volume. Ventricular arrhythmias may occur in the presence of increased catecholamine levels and therefore adrenaline should be avoided or injected, slowly, in a very dilute solution during halothane administration. Halothane depresses skeletal, cardiac and uterine muscle and potentiates muscle relaxants. There is evidence that repeated halothane anaesthetics over a short period of time may sensitise the patient to halothane and lead to hepatic changes, known as 'halothane hepatitis'. Halothane should not be administered again until 6 months have elapsed since the previous exposure.

Enflurane
A volatile non-flammable liquid with a boiling point of 56.5°C. Induction and recovery are reasonably fast (blood/gas solubility coefficient 1.9) but it is not as potent as halothane (MAC 1.68%). An inhalational induction is therefore difficult with enflurane. It produces a dose-related depression of tidal volume, respiratory rate and myocardial contractility. Sensitisation of the myocardium to catecholamines is less than with halothane. Enflurane depresses skeletal, cardiac and uterine muscle and potentiates muscle relaxants. Metabolic products include inorganic fluoride, but the concentrations do not reach nephrotoxic levels. An abnormal EEG, similar to a seizure pattern, may occur at high concentrations and it is therefore not recommended for use in epileptic patients. Convulsions have followed its use. Enflurane does not appear to affect the normal liver.

Isoflurane
A volatile non-flammable liquid with a boiling point of 48.5°C. Induction and recovery are slightly faster than for halothane or enflurane (blood/gas solubility coefficient 1.4) and its potency lies between those of halothane and enflurane (MAC = 1.13%). Isoflurane is irritant to the airways with a pungent smell and therefore an inhalational induction with this agent is very difficult. The myocardium is not sensitised to catecholamines. Its depressant action on muscle is less than that of either halothane or enflurane. It also potentiates muscle relaxants. The inorganic fluoride production is about one-tenth that of enflurane (and therefore well below nephrotoxic potential) and no adverse effects on the liver have been reported. In normal clinical concentrations there is no effect on cerebral blood flow or intracranial pressure. Convulsions have followed its use.

Desflurane
This volatile agent was synthesised around the same time as
isoflurane, but has only recently found its way into clinical practice.
It is more volatile than any of the other agents (boiling point 23.5°C).
Onset and recovery are extremely rapid (blood/gas solubility
coefficient 0.42) although its potency is much less (MAC 6.1%).
It has a pungent smell which makes inhalational induction difficult.
There is no sensitisation of the myocardium to catecholamines and
no metabolic fluoride production. Its very fast offset is an advantage
in day-stay procedures. Unfortunately it is expensive and requires
a special heated vaporiser for delivery because of the proximity of
its boiling point to room temperature.

Sevoflurane
Although the most recent addition to the volatile agents available
in Europe, sevoflurane has been in use in Japan for some time.
It has a boiling point of 58.5°C, a blood/gas solubility coefficient of
0.6 and a MAC of 2.1% It therefore has a fairly rapid onset and this,
combined with its pleasant smell and lack of airway irritability,
makes it ideal for inhalational induction. It does not sensitise the
heart to catecholamines and it produces no harmful metabolites.
Some concern has been expressed that a potentially toxic
substance (compound A) may be produced from the interaction
between sevoflurane and soda lime. This has not, however, proved
to be a problem in clinical use, even at low fresh gas flows. Its
rapid recovery has given it a significant role in day-stay procedures.

TOTAL INTRAVENOUS ANAESTHESIA (TIVA)

The origins of anaesthesia lie in a technique by which induction
and maintenance of anaesthesia was achieved using the
inhalational route. With the introduction of intravenous agents
with rapid onset, the basic technique has evolved into one in
which intravenous agents are used for induction and inhalational
agents for maintenance. The introduction of sevoflurane has
brought inhalational induction back into everyday practice. The
availability of intravenous agents with a shorter duration of action
has allowed the technique of TIVA to develop.

    The technique of TIVA requires that all components of the
anaesthetic are given by the intravenous route. Many anaesthetists
do still use nitrous oxide, but, ideally, an air/oxygen mixture
should be used. The only intravenous agent presently suited to
TIVA is propofol and there is a wealth of data available concerning
this practice. Historically, Althesin was suitable for TIVA, and
eltanolone should also be so.

    There are a number of specific indications when TIVA is particularly
advantageous (Table 1.3). It is used in routine practice by many
anaesthetists, however, because of a widely held belief that recovery
is more rapid, especially for day cases and shorter surgical procedures.

The disadvantages are few (Table 1.3): the most problematic is the wide variation in pharmacokinetics which has led a number of anaesthetists to worry about the control of depth of anaesthesia.

The development of target-controlled infusions (TCI) has reduced that problem. The traditional technique of TIVA requires the anaesthetist to administer boluses of agent, or an infusion, and titrate to an observed end-point. Various algorithms exist to help (e.g. the 10:8:6 regime for propofol). The TCI pump is supplied with the age and weight of the patient. The anaesthetist then selects a target plasma concentration and the pump chooses the infusion rate which will be required. This system is presently only available for propofol.

PREOPERATIVE CONSIDERATIONS

Up to 50% of patients presenting for surgery have a pre-existing medical condition and a positive drug history can be obtained from up to 60%. For specific details concerning the medical assessment and preparation of patients and potential drug interactions the reader is referred to Chapter 2.

The rules of starvation

For morning surgery, patients normally take nothing by mouth from midnight prior to anaesthesia; for afternoon surgery, a light early breakfast (06.00 hours) is usually allowed. This regimen can put certain patients at risk, particularly the newborn or the diabetic patient, and intravenous fluids and nutrients should be given. It is also unpleasant for the patient. Recent evidence suggests that clear fluids (water or juice, not milky drinks) may be given to the elective surgical patient up to 2 hours preoperatively without compromising safety and this routine is becoming more common.

Urgent procedures in the unstarved patient present a dilemma and considerable debate has taken place as to whether the stomach of the patient at great risk should be emptied. The passage of a

Table 1.3   Total intravenous anaesthesia (TIVA)

Indications
When a volatile agent is inadvisable or contraindicated, e.g. malignant hyperthermia
To provide sedation during regional techniques
Surgery in the airway
Cardiopulmonary bypass
Anaesthesia 'in the field'
When 100% oxygen is required

Disadvantages
Need for a dedicated intravenous access
Need for an accurate infusion pump
Wide variation exists in the pharmacokinetics of intravenous agents

nasogastric tube may induce vomiting, although this in itself may be hazardous and most unpleasant. Unless the tube is of a very large size it will not facilitate the complete emptying of the stomach. Apomorphine, an emetic, has been used, but this also is unpleasant. Metoclopramide is an agent that does speed the emptying of the stomach although doubt has been expressed as to its effectiveness in the acutely ill or trauma patient and it does requires time to work.

Current teaching does not advocate active emptying of the stomach (except for the use of metoclopramide) but relies upon waiting as long as possible and then using a rapid sequence induction technique with cricoid pressure and tracheal intubation.

Premedication

Premedicant drugs serve many purposes, particularly control of secretions, alleviation of anxiety and production of a foundation on which to construct the anaesthetic.

Atropine, hyoscine and glycopyrrolate are used as anti-sialogogues. Their desirability in premedication is debatable. A dry mouth is uncomfortable and more likely to be traumatised. Surgery in and around the mouth and airway may, however, be facilitated by a reduction in secretions. Atropine has been associated with a fall in oxygen saturation and hyoscine can produce confusion in the elderly. Glycopyrollate does not cross the blood–brain barrier.

Although anxiolytic agents may appear ideal, they have been shown to produce a significant fall in arterial oxygen tension and should therefore not be given to those patients with limited cardiorespiratory reserve. Similarly opioid premedication may be associated with respiratory depression. A preoperative visit by the anaesthetist has anxiolytic properties, is efficacious and has no adverse side-effects.

There are a number of considerations which are relevant. Amnesia is valuable if there is a significant emotional component present. Analgesia might be required if pain exists preoperatively and also the use of a long-acting agent will produce analgesia throughout surgery and into the postoperative period. Antibiotic prophylaxis should be considered if the patient has an artificial implant or a condition which can predispose to bacterial endocarditis. An antacid or H_2 receptor antagonist should be considered in the at-risk patient. Finally, the need for prophylaxis against venous thrombroembolic disease should be considered.

ADMINISTRATION OF ANAESTHESIA

Induction of anaesthesia is generally secured by intravenous injection of the chosen induction agent. Care must be taken to avoid intra-arterial injection, or extravascular injection. The risk of intra-arterial injection, though much reduced, is still present if a vein on the back of the hand is used.

Inhalational induction employs either oxygen-enriched air or nitrous oxide and oxygen as carrier agents. To be a useful induction agent, a volatile anaesthetic agent requires a high vapour pressure at room temperature. In addition, a low blood/gas solubility coefficient and a low MAC value (e.g. halothane 2.3 and 0.75 sevoflurane 0.6 and 2.1 respectively) are desirable. The tidal ventilation alone is commonly used to carry the vapour, originally from an open system (e.g. Schimmelbusch mask), or from a draw-over apparatus, such as the EMO (Epstein MacIntosh Oxford) vaporiser. Spontaneous ventilation from a high-flow circuit or taking several maximum inspirations from a pre-filled circuit are presently the common techniques.

Drugs which produce general anaesthesia usually also produce respiratory and cardiovascular depression. Patients with limited respiratory or cardiovascular reserve are therefore particularly at risk.

If an inhalational induction is used the pulmonary ventilation and the cardiac output will influence the rate at which the anaesthetic agent is taken up, and hence the time to induce anaesthesia. The rate of induction is directly related to the alveolar minute volume and inversely related to the cardiac output. The use of an intravenous induction agent may circumvent the ventilatory and circulatory factors, but on the other hand may cause cardiovascular and respiratory depression, thereby not only affecting the subsequent introduction of inhalational agents, but in some circumstances could jeopardise basic gas exchange.

The basic but essential concepts upon which the administration of every anaesthetic must be constructed are depicted in Figures 1.2 and 1.3. These may be summarised as follows:

1. Protection of alveolar ventilation and oxygenation

a. Control the patency of the airway. Obstruction of the airway leads to a cessation of air flow and hence of alveolar ventilation. The patency of the airway may be ensured by the simple expedient of holding the lower jaw forward (not by closing the mouth), intubation, or the insertion of an oropharyngeal airway, nasopharyngeal airway or a laryngeal mask airway.

b. Maintain adequate tidal volume (V_T) and frequency (f) with limitation of the apparatus dead space (V_D) or provision for carbon dioxide absorption. The fractional content of gases inhaled may be varied as required, but breathing is essential for alveolar ventilation and, in the presence of respiratory depression, the adequacy of alveolar ventilation must be ensured by controlling the tidal volume and ventilatory frequency. Apparatus dead space should be reduced to a minimum to reduce re-breathing of expired alveolar gas.

c. Provision of an effective oxygen concentration (F_1O_2) in the gas and anaesthetic mixture from the anaesthetic machine.

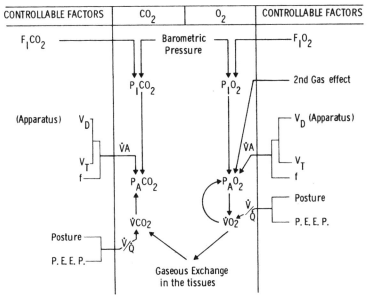

Fig 1.2 Factors influencing gaseous exchange in the respiratory system.

2. Protection of oxygen delivery to the tissues

a. Correct any deficiency in haemoglobin concentration by blood transfusion (not necessarily if the patient has a chronic anaemia, e.g. renal disease–see Chapter 2). Desaturation and anaemia can result in a dangerous fall in the amount of oxygen available to the tissues. These can only be compensated for by increasing the cardiac output through an increase in cardiac work.

b. Maintenance and/or correction of blood volume. Perfusion can only be maintained if venous return, and therefore cardiac output, is maintained.

c. Assess adequacy of cardiac output and where necessary support with inotropic and/or chronotropic agents. Maintain heart rate > 40 and < 120 per minute.

d. Control of peripheral resistance. Vasoconstriction leads to reduced tissue perfusion and a greater afterload puts extra strain on the heart.

AWARENESS

'Balanced anaesthesia' using muscle relaxants and small doses of hypnotic and analgesic agents is a very common technique at present. It may, however, be associated with an increased incidence of awareness during surgery. This is particularly the case in the patient who has received no premedication and only nitrous oxide with a

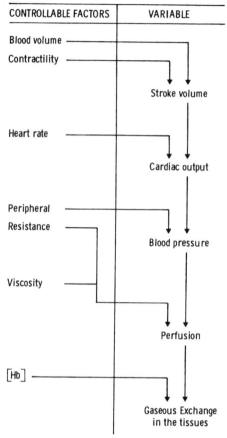

Fig 1.3 Factors influencing gaseous exchange in the cardiovascular system.

muscle relaxant. The addition of opioids, volatile agents and dissociative agents reduces this possibility.

MONITORING

The original anaesthetic monitoring system consisted of the anaesthetist's eyes and fingers. The value of these should not be underestimated and they should still be used during every anaesthetic in addition to those monitors resulting from modern technological advances. Minimal monitoring standards vary slightly between countries but generally consist of pulse oximeter, continous ECG and regular non-invasive blood pressure. These should be attached before anaesthesia is induced and continue until after the patient has regained consciousness.

In addition to the minimum monitoring standard referred to above, inspired oxygen fraction and tidal carbon dioxide concentration and volatile agent concentration should also be available. If the anaesthetic technique requires intermittent positive pressure ventilation, airway pressure and minute volume (or tidal volume and rate) are required. If a muscle relaxant is in use, a nerve stimulator should be attached. For prolonged surgery or an at-risk patient, core temperature should be added to the above.

In cases of more complex surgery, or for the high-risk patient, a central venous pressure line, an arterial line or even a pulmonary artery flotation catheter may be required. A urinary catheter may be inserted to allow measurement of urine output to help to maintain more accurate fluid balance overall.

POSTOPERATIVE CARE

Two aspects of postoperative care that principally concern anaesthetists are pain relief and oxygenation. Pain relief is dealt with in Chapter 4.

Drugs administered pre-, intra- and postoperatively may contribute to postoperative hypoxaemia. The anaesthetist and surgeon should therefore both have rapid access to the patient in the immediate postoperative period and a high nurse/patient ratio is mandatory. Many analgesics cause respiratory depression, but so can inadequate analgesia, particularly following abdominal surgery.

Hypoxaemia is more likely in the elderly, and also after thoracic and upper abdominal surgery. A reduction in functional residual capacity and the loss of the pulmonary vasoconstrictor response to hypoxia caused by anaesthetic agents are thought to be major contributory factors. Oxygen masks should be used routinely for those at risk, but oxygen therapy alone should not be used to compensate for respiratory depression. Respiratory stimulants such as doxapram may have a place, but these will not overcome inadequate reversal of non-depolarising muscle-relaxants and should be used with great care in patients with hypertension or tachycardia. If in doubt, re-intubate the trachea to guarantee the safety of the patient and then the situation can be appraised with less urgency.

Posture was thought to be an important factor in postoperative hypoxaemia, i.e. sitting is better than lying, but recent work has cast doubt on this view. A semirecumbent position may, nevertheless, assist respiratory function in patients who are obese or who have increased intra-abdominal pressure. Good pain relief certainly helps the patient but may not improve oxygenation; airway obstruction is probably the commonest cause of severe acute hypoxaemia and should always be avoided. Shivering and increased muscle tone can also lead to hypoxaemia. Maintenance of cardiac output by correct fluid mangement and the avoidance of myocardial depressants also minimises hypoxaemia.

ANAESTHESIA IN THE NEONATE
Airway management
As a general rule, anaesthesia in the neonate should only be attempted by those suitably skilled and who undertake anaesthesia in neonates and infants on a regular basis. There is a marked difference in the anatomy of the airway, making intubation more difficult. The larynx is positioned rather more anteriorly than in the adult and higher, under the posterior aspect of the tongue. Laryngoscopy is usually achieved best by using a straight-bladed laryngoscope, the blade being placed behind the V-shaped epiglottis. The epiglottis is flattened by the blade, allowing the glottic opening to be seen. Laryngoscopy is hindered further by the relatively large neonatal head which causes anterior neck flexion, leading to soft tissue obstructing the view of the glottis. This may be overcome by placing a small pillow behind the shoulders, the head being supported at a lower level, thereby extending the neck over the pillow. It is important to secure the endotracheal tube in three planes so as to reduce movement, and therefore laryngeal trauma, to a minimum. For this reason nasal intubation is frequently used, particularly if prolonged ventilation is anticipated. A cuffed endotracheal tube, which would reduce the diameter of the airway, increasing the resistance to airflow, is not used. For positive pressure ventilation an airtight fit is achieved between the walls of the larynx and the tube in the region of the cricoid cartilage, the narrowest part of the neonatal larynx.

The apparatus dead space must be reduced to a minimum. Even a few millilitres of apparatus dead space, which may be no hazard in an adult, may markedly reduce the alveolar ventilation when the tidal volume is only 20 ml, the physiological dead space 5 ml and the minute ventilation about 400 ml (2.5 kg neonate).

Heat loss
The surface area of a neonate is much greater relative to its body weight than that of an adult. This, together with a higher skin temperature, may lead to excessive heat loss. Loss of heat combined with an immature temperature-regulating centre may, in a cold environment, lead to a fall in temperature. As body temperature falls, hyperkalaemia, hyperglycaemia and acidosis result. It is essential therefore to monitor the body temperature, using an oesophageal or rectal thermometer, and to reduce heat loss during anaesthesia and surgery of the neonate by the use of a warmed operating theatre, constant body-temperature blankets, cotton wool insulation and aluminium foil. Heated blankets must not exceed 42°C.

Monitoring
Laboratory assessment of plasma sodium, potassium, chloride, glucose, protein and urea may be valuable for monitoring electrolyte

imbalance, dehydration and the response to treatment. The blood urea may rise markedly in postmature babies and may vary considerably with pyrexia and marginal dehydration. The neonatal kidney may not be able to cope with a sodium load and therefore it is important in planning the intravenous fluid regime to avoid administering a sodium overload during and after surgery. A 5% dextrose solution may be all that is required. It is important to remember that when prolonged gastric secretion or vomiting has occurred sodium and chloride replacement may be necessary. The neonate also excretes potassium less efficiently than the adult, and indeed the plasma concentration of potassium may be considerably raised following surgery. The calcium requirement is generally met by the milk diet, but in the presence of severe diarrhoea calcium may need to be supplemented intravenously if it is shown to be necessary. The magnesium requirement is not usually a matter for concern, though in the presence of faecal fistula or an ileostomy, magnesium replacement may be required.

Fluid replacement
Total body water and extracellular water constitute higher proportions of the total body weight in the neonate than in the adult. Insensible loss generally amounts to 100 ml per day and this volume in addition to the volume of urine produced should be replaced. However, when the neonate is nursed in an incubator with an atmospheric humidity approaching 100%, insensible fluid loss may be halved. Urine output increases from approximately 20 ml on the second day of life to 150 ml on the seventh day. The neonate's initial blood volume is dependent upon transfer from the placenta. The initial haemoglobin value is approximately 20 g.dl^{-1}; and this is reduced progressively by haemolysis. The fall in value is most rapid during the first 2 weeks of life and at 3 months the value has usually fallen to about 10 g.dl^{-1}. The maintenance of blood volume is of major importance, and blood loss must be measured, by weighing of swabs or by a colorimetric method. Loss should be replaced with whole blood when loss of 10% total blood volume approaches.

Anaesthesia
Preoperative assessment should include weight, temperature, respiratory and cardiovascular status and the presence of twitching (hypocalcaemia, hypoglycaemia, hypoxia). Atropine 0.15 mg is normally given as premedication with vitamin K if the infant is less than 3 days old. It was believed for many years that general anaesthesia was not required for intubation of the neonate. Current teaching advises against that approach if possible and, as in older babies, either an inhalation or intravenous induction may be used. The thoracic cage is very pliable and this may lead to a marked reduction in the pulmonary functional residual capacity, and therefore hypoxia with cyanosis may occur very rapidly when

ventilation is interrupted. This effect is further augmented by the relatively higher pulmonary vascular resistance and an initial right-to-left shunt. Spontaneous ventilation in the neonate depends largely on the diaphragm. Rib excursion is limited by the horizontal position at rest and by the distortion resulting from diaphragmatic contraction. Ventilation is normally controlled using a muscle relaxant and is monitored using an oesophageal or praecordial stethoscope. The most commonly used breathing system is the T-piece. For spontaneous ventilation a gas flow of three times the minute ventilation prevents CO_2 retention. The Rees modification (reservoir bag with through-flow) facilitates controlled ventilation. Higher flows are used to prevent CO_2 retention (3–4 l. min^{-1}).

Surgery

There are several conditions that need urgent surgical intervention in the first two months of life. These include:

1. Pyloric stenosis
2. Exomphalos
3. Gastroschisis
4. Tracheo-oesophageal fistula
5. Congenital diaphragmatic hernia
6. Congenital cystic disease of lung
7. Developmental abnormalities of spine and cranium
8. Hydrocephalus (insertion of pressure relief valve)

The detailed management of these conditions cannot be covered adequately in a book of this nature, but the fundamental concepts of managing the newborn remain the same. Anaesthesia for some of these conditions is covered in Chapter 3.

ANAESTHESIA IN THE ELDERLY

The two limits of life, i.e. the neonate and the elderly, in some ways reflect each other. The elderly patient is generally more fragile than the younger adult. Fragile skin and blood vessels lead to more rapid bruising and brittle bones are more likely to fracture.

Advanced degenerative diseases—cardiac, pulmonary, vascular, cerebrovascular, renal and hepatic—may be present. In addition, frank cardiopulmonary disease, low-grade chronic renal and pulmonary infection and muscle wasting, frequently associated with malnutrition, and anaemia, make anaesthesia and surgery more hazardous in the elderly and dictate the need for the most careful preoperative assessment.

Degenerative processes reduce the functional reserve of all systems, and therefore the onset of disease in a system already damaged by a degenerative process is more likely to lead to complete system failure. The elderly with arteriosclerosis are less tolerant of hypoxaemia, particularly in low flow states or if the perfusion pressure is inadequate.

Cardiac failure is common in the elderly and is often associated with coronary artery disease, loss of muscle volume and coronary blood vessel occlusion. Arteriosclerosis affecting the aortic valve and aorta may limit the cardiac output. The elderly therefore have an impaired myocardial reserve and may not be able to adjust to sudden changes in blood volume, hypothermia or hyperthermia, to the negative inotropic effects of anaesthetic drugs, to active diseases (including sepsis), or to increased metabolic demands following surgery.

The elderly lungs are also subject to degenerative changes. Airway closure occurs when the intrapleural pressure (dependent on gravity and the volume of the chest) exceeds the critical closing pressure (dependent on elastic recoil) and thus in the elderly, in whom elastic tissue has been lost, airway closure occurs at a higher lung volume. When closing volume exceeds the functional residual capacity, airway closure takes place during normal tidal flow. The relation between age and closing volume is as follows:

Closing volume (% of total lung capacity) = 19.4 + 0.5 (age)

At 65 years the closing volume exceeds the FRC when standing, and there is therefore inefficient gas mixing and P_aO_2 falls.

Pulmonary changes in disease usually lead to either increased airway resistance (obstructive) or reduced pulmonary excursion (restrictive) and associated pulmonary vascular disease. Chronic bronchitis and emphysema are the most common presentations. The presence of pulmonary fibrosis or neoplasia and associated intrathoracic disease, including a pleural effusion, must, however, be considered. A careful assessment of pulmonary and cardiovascular function is vital. Preoperative preparation to improve breathing and reduce infection is essential in all but emergency situations. Blood transfusion, fluid and electrolyte therapy may be required to correct anaemia, dehydration and electrolyte imbalance. Anaesthesia should be instituted and maintained in such a way that further impairment of cardiovascular compensation is reduced to a minimum. Intermittent positive pressure ventilation may be required to ensure adequate oxygenation and the prevention of hypercarbia. Heat loss should also be reduced to a minimum. Confusion is not uncommon in the elderly and may have many causes. However, it may be precipitated by sedative or anxiolytic drugs, including hyoscine.

Local anaesthetic techniques have been shown to have advantages over general anaesthesia in the elderly—the morbidity and mortality associated with spinal anaesthesia being less for hip surgery than with general anaesthesia. It is advisable to avoid the sympathetic blockade associated with higher blocks because of the obtunded vasomotor responses in the elderly. Local anaesthesia, whether spinal or epidural, spreads higher in the elderly, and thus volumes of local anaesthetics should be modified accordingly. Early postoperative mobility is essential.

ANAESTHESIA IN PREGNANCY

FIRST TRIMESTER

It is wise to avoid the administration of any drug during the early part of pregnancy. The reasons are the risks of teratogenicity and spontaneous miscarriage. However, there is no evidence to suggest that the administration of a general anaesthetic carries a specific teratogenic risk because the only evidence available relates to prolonged exposure in animals. A further confounding issue is that arguably the most hazardous time is when the mother herself may not realise that she is pregnant.

SECOND TRIMESTER

Miscarriage may be associated with general anaesthesia, particularly if intra-abdominal surgery is performed. If surgery is essential, the second trimester is generally regarded as safer than the first.

THIRD TRIMESTER

Supine hypotension
The uterus may, if the patient lies supine, obstruct the inferior vena cava and thereby impair venous return. The resultant fall in cardiac output may lead to severe hypotension. The incidence of this can be reduced by tilting the patient to the left. Supine hypotension only occurs in a minority of patients and these patients are thought to lack collateral vessels bypassing the inferior vena cava. Aortic compression may also add to the reduction in placental perfusion caused by the hypotension.

Increased acid secretion
The dangers of gastric acid inhalation (described by Mendelson in 1945) have been well documented. It is not always possible to plan anaesthesia in pregnancy and patients may therefore have had a recent meal. Furthermore, gastric emptying is slowed and, owing to the distortion of the diaphragm caused by the large uterus, the cardia may be less effective in preventing regurgitation. Regurgitation and inhalation of gastric contents may therefore occur. This likelihood must be reduced. In the first instance the pH of the stomach contents may be raised by oral antacids (30 ml of 0.3 molar sodium citrate solution is the present antacid of choice). Ranitidine may also be given. Direct stomach emptying with a gastro-oesophageal tube is not normally considered necessary, neither is the use of apomorphine. Atropine is now thought to reduce the tone of the gastro-oesophageal sphincter and glycopyrollate has been reported to raise the pH of the gastric contents.

Preoxygenation before induction of anaesthesia will obviate the need for positive pressure oxygenation using a face mask which may encourage gastric emptying by squeezing the stomach between the diaphragm and the other abdominal contents, including the large uterus. Cricoid pressure should be applied to prevent regurgitation into the oropharynx during induction.

Fetal gas exchange

Gas exchange between maternal and fetal blood takes place in the placenta. The umbilical artery blood gas tensions are 2 kPa P_{O_2} and 6 kPa P_{CO_2}. These values are altered to 4 kPa P_{O_2} and 5.5 kPa P_{CO_2} in the umbilical vein as a result of the oxygen and carbon dioxide gradients which exist between the fetal and maternal blood.

The double Bohr effect facilitates oxygen transfer to the fetus. The transfer of fetal carbon dioxide to the maternal circulation moves the maternal oxygen haemoglobin saturation curve to the right, thereby reducing the affinity of maternal haemoglobin for oxygen which releases oxygen. On the other hand, the rapid transfer of carbon dioxide across the membrane increases the affinity of fetal haemoglobin for oxygen, thereby facilitating the transfer of oxygen across the placental membrane.

A similar mechanism facilitates carbon dioxide transfer to the mother—the double Haldane effect—but is not quite so effective because of low levels of carbonic anhydrase in the fetus.

Cardiovascular changes during pregnancy

A marked increase in cardiac output (30–40%) may occur in association with a rise in blood volume (50%), salt and water retention, and a fall in the haemoglobin concentration. Retraction of the uterus after delivery may therefore produce a major fluid overload. The vasoconstricting effect of ergometrine is undesirable and synthetic oxytocin is to be preferred.

Effects of drugs on the uterus and fetus

In general terms a high concentration of anaesthetic, analgesic and sedative drugs will depress uterine contractions. It is therefore important to use drugs in the minimum effective therapeutic dose. Any of the volatile agents can be used safely in low concentrations. Thiopentone is similarly unlikely to affect uterine muscle tone if normal sleep doses are used. Indeed, the effect of thiopentone on the fetus is likely to be of greater importance than its effect on the uterus. Ketamine disobeys the general rule and is reported to increase uterine muscle tone. Narcotic agents, when used in normal therapeutic doses, are unlikely to affect uterine contractions and can be used safely. However, in higher doses, uterine and fetal depression may occur.

Drug transfer to the fetus across the placenta depends on its lipid solubility, its degree of ionisation and its protein-binding properties, as with any other membrane. It also depends on the timing of the injection and on whether the patient is in labour. A drug injected just prior to a contraction may not reach the placenta at all. Detoxification of drugs may occur in the placenta as amine oxidases and esterases are present. There is no evidence to suggest that benzodiazepines have a deleterious effect on the fetus although diazepam and lorazepam have both been reported to be associated with low APGAR scores at birth.

2. Problems associated with medical disease processes

While there are innumerable diseases, their gross physiological effects are limited and not all of these are of relevance to anaesthesia.

The following catalogues the physiological/pharmacological disturbances of relevance to anaesthesia:

- Drug interactions
- Acute adverse reactions to drugs
- Altered sensitivity to drugs
- Upper airway problems
- Lower airway problems
- Failure of oxygenation (respiratory)
- Critical ventilatory ability
- High cardiac output
- Fixed cardiac output
- Low cardiac output
- Failure of oxygenation (cardiovascular)
- Abnormal vasomotor control
- Reduced oxygen carriage
- Increased risk of thrombosis
- Increased risk of haemolysis
- Disorder of haemostasis
- Reduced ability to cooperate
- Increased risk of cerebral damage
- Altered metabolic state
- Australia antigen and HIV
- Increased risk of renal failure
- Skeletal disease
- Skin and mucous membranes at risk

INTERACTIONS BETWEEN THERAPEUTIC AGENTS AND AGENTS USED IN ANAESTHESIA

Antacids

Sodium bicarbonate
In excess, this may cause systemic alkalosis, thereby influencing the effect, duration and excretion of other ionised drugs.

Antibiotics
The following antibiotics have been shown to interfere to various degrees with neuromuscular transmission:

Amikacin	Gentamycin	Polymyxin B
Bacitracin	Kanamycin	Streptomycin
Clindamycin	Lincomycin	Tobramycin
Colistin/colymycin	Neomycin	Tetracyclines

Anticholinesterases

Ecothiopate iodide eye drops
Ecothiopate, a non-reversible anticholinesterase, may prolong the action of suxamethonium.

Antidepressants

Tricyclics
Noradrenaline re-uptake is inhibited by these drugs. They may cause potentiation of sedatives and sympathomimetic agents, the latter leading to hypertension: adrenaline and noradrenaline are absolutely contraindicated.

There is evidence that the 'tricyclics' increase the incidence of arrhythmias during halothane anaesthesia.

Monoamine oxidase inhibitors
The inhibition of monoamine oxidase (MAO) leads to the accumulation of 5HT, dopamine and noradrenaline within the neuron, and interaction with the following:
- Tricyclic antidepressants
- Sympathomimetic amines, levodopa, pethidine, morphine and other narcotic analgesics
- Pentazocine, Phenazocine

Therapy must discontinued for at least three weeks preoperatively if these agents are to be given.

Lithium
Sodium imbalance may occur. Toxic levels can potentiate barbiturates and prolong the response to neuromuscular blocking agents and reduce the required dose of intravenous and inhaled anaesthetic agents, may cause hypotension, dysrhythmias, A V block. Convulsions have been reported.

Antihypertensives
Some may obtund the normal cardiovascular reflexes and increase the sensitivity to general anaesthetic agents, e.g. hydrallazine, methyldopa, reserpine and guanethidine.

Beta adrenergic receptor blockers are reported to induce a myasthenic syndrome and to unmask myasthenia gravis.

Trimetaphan may potentiate the neuromuscular blocking action of both non-depolarisers and depolarisers.

Nitroglycerine prolongs the effect of pancuronium.

Care should be taken with sympathomimetic agents if the patient is taking debrisoquine or guanethidine.

Anti-Parkinson therapy

Parkinson's disease is a degenerative condition of the CNS—
destruction of the dopamine-containing cells in the basal ganglia.

Amantidine

Care should be taken with concurrent administration of central
nervous system stimulants.

Levodopa

Levodopa, the precursor of dopamine, may interact with other
drugs. However, during normal anaesthesia there should be few
problems, although, because beta adrenergic receptors in the heart
are stimulated there is a reduction in noradrenaline stores in the
myocardium. An increased incidence of arrhythmias under
halothane anaesthesia has been noted. Care should be taken
during administration of antihypertensives or sympathomimetics.

Patients undergoing general anaesthesia should have therapy
stopped the night before operation. MAO-B inhibitors may inhibit
dopamine metabolism and increase dopamine activity. Pethidine
may result in a hypertensive crisis. Note there are MAO-A and
MAO-B subtypes. Selegiline (MAO-B) is used in combination with
levodopa to prevent the progressive reduction of levodopa effect.

Methixine

Blood pressure may be unstable as there is the possibility of
autonomic lability. Other useful drugs include carbidopa which
reduces the dose of levodopa needed.

Beta adrenergic receptor blockers

Cardio-selective

- Practolol
- Metoprolol
- Atenolol

Non-selective

- Propranolol
- Oxprenolol
- Labetolol

Heart failure can be precipitated by beta
adrenergic receptor blockade and bradycardia
and may limit the heart's ability to respond to
large changes in blood volume and/or
peripheral resistance.

Care should be taken with all general anaesthetic agents.

Carbenoxolone

Hypokalaemia, sodium and water retention may exacerbate
hypertension, cardiac failure, oedema and muscle weakness and
alter the action of some drugs such as digitalis.

Contraceptive pill

Increased risk of deep vein thrombosis.

Digitalis glycosides

Digitalis intoxication—atrio-ventricular block, extra systoles, nausea and vomiting—may be precipitated by electrolyte disorders and drugs. Hypokalaemia, hypomagnesaemia, hypernatraemia, hypercalcaemia and alkalosis. Diuretics can cause hypokalaemia, as do carbenoxolone, the contraceptive pill, corticosteroids, reserpine and catecholamines.

Diuretics

Potassium-sparing (amiloride, triamterene, spironolactone)
A relative hypovolaemia may exist, and may be revealed if a vasodilator agent is administered.

Non-potassium-sparing (frusemide, bumetanide, piretanide, ethacrynic acid)
Hypokalaemia and hypovolaemia may develop.

Endocrine therapy

Glucocorticoids
Steroid supplementation may be necessary.

Mineralocorticoid
Check electrolyte homeostasis and fluid balance.

Insulin
Abnormal potassium levels may develop and change the actions of other agents. Thus we must confirm the potassium concentration. Potassium changes normally only occur if an acute diabetic state is being treated.

Pitressin
Check electrolyte homeostasis and fluid balance.

ACUTE ADVERSE REACTIONS TO DRUGS

Induction agents

Acute adverse reactions must be differentiated from the effects of relative overdosage or an exaggerated response to the drug. Features of acute adverse reaction to intravenous induction agents: life-threatening features are bronchospasm, cardiovascular collapse, oedema of the airway; non-life-threatening features are erythema, rashes and urticaria.

Causes
- Mast cells bind to IgE, releasing histamine ⎫ Anaphylactoid
- Activation of C3 complement ⎭
- Immune mediated mechanism   Anaphylactic

(An anaphylactic reaction requires previous exposure to the agent.)

Failure to report reactions to drugs makes it difficult to assess their incidence. Reactions to Althesin, for example, were estimated to range from 1 in 9 to 1 in 19.

Management of the acute major adverse reaction
1. Administer oxygen—intubation may be necessary and IPPV
2. Set up an intravenous infusion—give fluids if hypotensive
3. i.v. adrenaline for bronchospasm
4. H_1, and H_2 antagonists
5. Hydrocortisone
6. Monitor the ECG

All barbiturates are absolutely contraindicated for patients with porphyria—a disease due to defect in haem synthesis. Their use may result in lower motor neuron paralysis, psychic disturbances, abdominal pain, tachycardia, hypertension or possibly death. Etomidate and propofol are also contraindicated in porphyria, but ketamine is considered safe. Halothane, opioids and muscle relaxants are safe but pancuronium and lignocaine should be avoided.

Neuromuscular blocking drugs
Histamine can be released by both non-depolarising and depolarising agents. If severe, the reaction should be considered to be an anaphyactoid reaction and treated as above. The most dramatic and life-threatening reaction following the injection of a muscle relaxant is malignant hyperpyrexia in response to the injection of suxamethonium.

Malignant hyperpyrexia (MH)
Incidence — approximately 1:200 000 in the UK
       — MH may not be induced on first exposure to drugs known to induce it (44% probability)
       — greater in patients undergoing surgery for hernia, squint and spinal deformity
       — most patients are of late childhood/early adult age
Inherited — autosomal dominant with variable expression
Induced by— all volatile anaesthetic agents
       — suxamethonium
       — stress—the unknown factor—the absence of this may be responsible for the 56% chance that MH will not be induced in those known to be susceptible
Indicators — muscle spasm
       — inappropriate tachycardia
       — tachypnoea
       — cyanosis
       — oozing—disseminated intravascular coagulation (DIC)
       — Arrhythmias, cardiac arrest

Management
Diagnosis — a temperature rise of > 1°C per 10 minutes
(exclude other causes of pyrexia—infection, atropine
overdose, warm environment)
— muscle spasm (exclude other causes—dystrophia
myotonia, myotonia congenita)
Discontinue inhalational agents and surgery.
Hyperventilate with 100% oxygen.
Set up intravenous infusion:
- $NaHCO_3$: 100 mmol to reduce acidosis
- 10% dextrose and 20 units soluble insulin—to lower $[K^+]$

Take arterial blood sample for acid/base and electrolyte analysis,
clotting 'screen' and $[Ca^{++}]$. Dantrolene, 1 $mg.kg^{-1}$
intravenously—this may need to be repeated after 5 min
(maximum dose 10 $mg.kg^{-1}$). Dantrolene may raise the plasma
potassium.
Methylprednisolone, dexamethasone, or hydrocortisone high dose.
Active cooling may be necessary:
- droperidol may aid cooling and reduce muscle spasm
- ice packs in groins, axillae and around the neck
- cool intravenous fluids
- cold water sponging and enhanced evaporation with fans
- peritoneal dialysis with cold fluid may be used

Catheterise the patient—save a urine sample for myoglobin analysis.
Mannitol 1 $g.kg^{-1}$ i.v. may protect against cerebral oedema and
renal failure.
Inotropic agents may be required to maintain the cardiac output.
Beta adrenergic receptor blockers may be required to treat
extrasystoles or tachyarrhythmias.
Recovery may be prolonged over several days during which
fluid and electrolyte balance must be continuously assessed and
adjusted. An osmotic diuresis should be maintained, and
potassium supplementation will be required. Further dantrolene
may be needed, 1–2 $mg.kg^{-1}$ four times a day.
The patient and relations should be subsequently investigated
by muscle biopsy.

Anaesthesia for the patient susceptible to MH
1. A vaporiser-free anaesthetic machine
2. Monitor of ECG, $F_{ET}CO_2$, S_pO_2, BP, temperature, establish access
for arterial blood analysis
3. Means for cooling should be at hand
4. Safe drugs:

Diazepam, droperidol	— premedication
Thiopentine, propofol, ketamine	— induction
50% nitrous oxide in oxygen	— maintenance
Pancuronium	

(Do **NOT** reverse neuromuscular blockade with neostigmine and atropine.)
Local anaesthetic agents may be used—procaine, tetracaine, lignocaine, bupivacaine and prilocaine are considered safe.
Mortality from MH is about 50%

Inhalational agents
All inhalational agents apart from nitrous oxide have been implicated in the genesis of malignant hyperpyrexia. Other acute adverse reactions are those associated with irritancy or acute affects of high dose: hypotension, laryngeal spasm, coughing, breath-holding, bronchospasm and hiccup. The correct management—turn the agent off and continue anaesthesia using i.v. agents.

Arrhythmias (p. 47) may occur spontaneously but are more likely in association with hypoxia or hypercarbia. Continuous monitoring of cardiac rhythm is essential.

RESPIRATORY DISEASE

Anaesthetic problems concern varying levels of ventilatory failure with or without associated cardiovascular decompensation, e.g.:
* Right ventricular hypertrophy/failure (cor pulmonale)
* Polycythaemia secondary to chronic hypoxia

UPPER AIRWAY PROBLEMS

Disease leads to:
CNS depression
Trauma
Infection   Patients in danger of
Tumour   spontaneous obstruction
Anatomical variations

Trismus   Patients less likely to be obstruct
Scleroderma   spontaneously but there may be
Burns   problems of oral endotracheal intubation

General approach to the patient with potential airway obstruction
Heavy sedation undesirable. Integrity of the airway is at risk in the unconscious. Consider using a naso-pharyngeal airway. Nurse in the lateral position when necessary to facilitate spontaneous breathing, drainage of secretions, or blood, in cases of trauma.

Problems
It is essential to assess the airway carefully, whether the patient to be anaesthetised is to breathe spontaneously or to be ventilated.

Management
1. Is endotracheal intubation necessary?
   a. to protect the airway
   b. to facilitate surgery
   c. to allow IPPV
If not, use another technique.
2. Assess the problem:
   a. Nature and size of lesion
   b. Severity of functional problem, e.g. can a laryngeal mask airway (LMA) be introduced, can a gas-tight fit be made between face and face mask?

In those with cervical or temporomandibular joint arthritis, ankylosis, or an abnormal jaw, a lateral X-ray of mandible and cervical spine (in extension and flexion) is necessary. (Fig. 2.1) Carry out indirect laryngoscopy. Consider awake fibreoptic laryngoscopy and intubation.
3. Premedication—**NONE** or only a light anxiolytic/neurolept premedication.
4. Preoxygenation. The body oxygen store of an adult male in normal respiratory health breathing air is approximately 1500 ml.

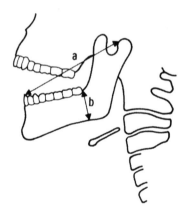

**If a/b = <3.6 intubation is
likely to be difficult**

Fig 2.1 Radiological measurements indicate likely difficult intubation. Also use Malampati test with the patient sitting, and tongue pushed forward and mouth wide open. Examine the anatomical features at the rear of the mouth. Clearly the more features that can be seen the more likely that intubation will be uncomplicated. Grades 1 and 2 do not usually present problems.
Grade 1   Uvula, soft palate, hard palate visible
Grade 2   Part of uvula, soft palate, hard palate visible
Grade 3   Soft palate, hard palate visible
Grade 4   Hard palate visible only

This can be increased three-fold by administering 100% oxygen for 3 minutes. If 3 minutes is too long to wait because of the urgency, then five or six deep breaths of 100% oxygen is almost as good.

5. Gaseous induction, with or without small i.v. dose of hypnotic agent.
   Deepen anaesthesia using halothane or sevoflurane or other inhalation agent with the patient breathing spontaneously.

6. Perform direct laryngoscopy as muscle relaxation occurs. Visualise the glottic opening.
   Do **NOT** use neuromuscular blocking agents until the indotracheal tube is in position.

7. Have stylets, bougies, various sizes of tubes and bronchoscopes available. Nasal intubation should be considered—it may be easier but may cause bleeding.

8. If intubation proves impossible, introduce LMA and continue. If less urgent, allow the patient to awaken and attempt intubation using local anaesthetic technique.

9. If still impossible, try trans-cricoid epidural needle technique.

10. Tracheotomy using local anaesthetic.

Success is enhanced by correct positioning of the patient, by maintaining oxygenation, by keeping the patient asleep when possible and by avoiding damage.

LOWER AIRWAY PROBLEMS

Disease leads to:
• Acute/chronic bronchitis
• Bronchospasm (asthma)
• Histamine release

Increased airway resistance may make ventilation difficult.

Chronic bronchitis/emphysema

Management: Severe respiratory dysfunction makes a regional anaesthetic technique advisable whenever possible. When this is impossible a controlled ventilation technique should be employed.

Preparation: Lung function tests.
$FEV_{1.0}$, P_aCO_2, P_aO_2.
Improve function by physiotherapy, antibiotics, antispasmodics and possibly mucolytics and steroids.

Premedication: Avoid opiates that may lead to respiratory depression and/or bronchospasm.

Induction: Pain, light anaesthesia, and irritant inhalational agents may induce bronchospasm. Histamine release may also occur.
Intravenous aminophylline (0.4–0.5 g) may be

administered slowly. Preoxygenate and then induce with an intravenous hypnotic and suxamethonium. Liberal 'topical' 4% lignocaine should be sprayed over the vocal cords and upper trachea before endotracheal intubation.

Maintenance: Neuromuscular blockade should be with cisatracurium, vecuronium or pancuronium and the ventilatory pattern should include a prolonged expiratory pause. Minute ventilation should be adjusted to compensate for the increased alveolar dead space. Adequate oxygenation should be ensured by the administration of 50:50 oxygen: nitrous oxide mixture and the depth of anaesthesia by halothane, isoflurane, sevoflurane or enflurane. Avoid desflurane (irritant).

Reversal: 1. Patients with an FEV < 1.0 litre and a P_aCO_2 > 5.3 kPa and a P_aO_2 < 8kPa breathing air should be electively ventilated with or without PEEP in the postoperative period.

2. Patients with an $FEV_{1.0}$ < 1.0 litre and normal blood gases and no excess bronchial secretions should be 'reversed' with neostigmine, after atropine or glycopyrollate graded oxygen therapy should be instituted.

Postoperative care: Conduction nerve block analgesia should be used rather than systemic analgesics.

Asthma

Assessment: Frequency of attacks and their control should be evaluated
Drug therapy—steroids—antispasmodics
Respiratory function tests
$FEV_{1.0}$ and the response to therapy
P_aCO_2, P_aO_2

Preparation: Physiotherapy
Antispasmodics
Inhalational therapy—IPPB with bronchodilators

Premedication: Anxiolytics
Bronchodilator—inhaler
Avoid opiates

Induction: Intravenous aminophylline may be given
Preoxygenation
Propofol, methohexitone or ketamine may be considered
(**AVOID** thiopentone)
Suxamethonium, vecuronium, pancuronium, cisatracurium or rocuronium
4% lignocaine spray to larynx and trachea

Maintenance:	Humidification
	IPPV
	PEEP may be helpful
	Inhalational agents other than desflurane may decrease bronchiolar tone if spasm is present
Reversal:	Use neostigmine with care
Postoperative care:	Graded oxygen therapy
	Conduction nerve block analgesia if suitable

FAILURE OF OXYGENATION

Causes:
$\dot{V}/\dot{Q}$ imbalance
Venous admixture
Chronic bronchitis/emphysema
Consolidation/collapse of lung
Pulmonary oedema
Vascular lung tumour
Hyaline membrane disease
Defects of heart and great vessels (see CVS subsection on p. 42)

Problems
Pulmonary shunting leads to deficient oxygenation and slows the uptake of inhalational agents. (Fig. 2.2)

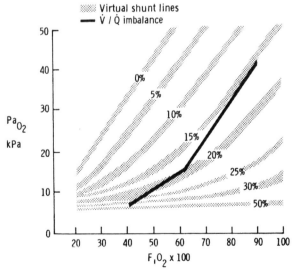

Fig 2.2 The relation between P_aCO_2 and F_iO_2 due to pulmonary shunt, i.e. $\dot{V}/\dot{Q}$ imbalance. One example shown.

Management
Use regional techniques where possible

Assessment: Alveolar–arterial (A–a) oxygen gradient
                P_aO_2 breathing air and oxygen
                P_aCO_2 breathing air and oxygen

Preparation: Aim to optimise pulmonary function with physiotherapy, antibiotics, antispasmodics, mucolytics

Premedication: Avoid respiratory depressants

Induction: Preoxygenation and denitrogenation to enhance the uptake of inhalational agents
An LA technique should be used where suitable

Maintenance: Avoid spontaneous ventilation as there is a tendency to underventilation which leads to further atelectasis and greater 'shunting'

Reversal: If endotracheal intubation employed, aspirate secretions from tracheo-bronchial tree. If preoperative $FEV_{1.0} < 1.0$ litre consider using a respiratory stimulant to maintain adequate alveolar ventilation (i.v. doxapram has been shown to be effective).

Postoperative: Physiotherapy to the chest and graded oxygen care
Avoid opiates if possible

EXCESSIVE PULMONARY SECRETIONS

Causes
- Chronic bronchitis
- Bronchiectasis
- Bronchopleural fistula (p. 95) lung abscess
- Pulmonary oedema
- Pneumonia
- Cholinergic poisoning (see p. 170)

Problems
Excess secretions occlude the smaller airways, making ventilation difficult. Infected secretions may contaminate the lung that is not infected.

Management
- Preoperative chest physiotherapy
- Treat infection
- Anti-sialogogues are best avoided, as secretions may become inspissated
- Endotracheal intubation and IPPV is preferable to a spontaneous ventilation technique (except for a bronchopleural fistula, see below).
- Frequent tracheal aspiration as required

- Endobronchial tubes are used to prevent flooding of the unaffected lung with purulent material or excess secretions in unilateral disease.
- Endobronchial tubes, see p. 186

Postoperative care
- Physiotherapy to the chest
- May be considered necessary to leave an endotracheal tube in situ, to facilitate the aspiration or clearance of secretions

CRITICAL VENTILATORY ABILITY

Inadequate spontaneous ventilation

Causes
- CNS depression
- Disease processes of the spinal cord (e.g. Guillain–Barré syndrome)
- Poliomyelitis
- Peripheral neuropathy
- Neuro-muscular disease
  — Myasthenia gravis
  — Myopathies
- Restricted movement of the chest wall
  — Crush injury of the chest
  — Obesity
- Acute lung disease
- Chronic lung disease
- Upper respiratory tract obstruction
- Diaphragmatic paralysis or immobility

Each of the above requires specific therapy but the functional problem of incipient respiratory failure needs a common approach when surgery is required.

Problems
Incipient respiratory failure (failure of oxygenation and/or failure of carbon dioxide excretion) can only be aggravated by anaesthesia and the decision to undertake surgery must be combined with a positive attitude to respiratory support during and after surgery.

Assessment
- Clinical history and examination
- Arterial blood gas measurement
- Pulmonary function tests (with exercise tolerance tests when possible)

Management
1. Elective ventilation
2. If ventilation is likely to be prolonged—tracheostomy
3. Chest physiotherapy

Inadequate ventilation with positive pressure ventilation

Causes
Massive leak:
• Bronchopleural fistula
• Tracheo-oesophageal fistula (TOF)

Problems
Both bronchopleural fistula and tracheo-oesophageal fistula are associated with pulmonary infection, the purulent material in the pleural space soiling the tracheobronchial tree in the former, and food or saliva in the latter. The larger the fistula the greater the soiling and also the greater the air leak should IPPV be instituted. On occasions the leak is so great that ventilation of the good lung is minimal.

Assessment
Bronchoscopy may indicate the site and the size of the fistula—but bronchoscopy itself is a hazardous procedure and should be carried out with the patient breathing spontaneously.

General approach
1. **NEVER** paralyse the patient before it is established that positive pressure ventilation can be effectively performed.
2. Isolation of fistula by use of appropriate endobronchial tube during spontaneous respiration.
3. Test isolation of leak by applying positive pressure to airway and assess leak into:
   a. underwater seal drain or
   b. into stomach.
4. If isolation of leak is complete then IPPV can be instituted.

   If inflation of the oesophagus via a TOF cannot be avoided then spontaneous respiration should be allowed until surgical access facilitates ligation of the fistula.
   When ventilating patients with bronchopleural fistula of a diffuse type, e.g. raw lung surface, ventilation may be achieved by using a conventional single-lumen tube, and a very short inspiratory phase. This ensures optimal distribution of gas throughout the lungs.

CARDIOVASCULAR DISEASE

Cardiovascular diseases may influence all other systems and thus present the anaesthetist with diverse problems e.g.:
1. Renal failure associated with hypertension
2. Intestinal stasis due to mesenteric embolisation
3. Cerebral ischaemia due to atheroma
4. Liver dysfunction due to right heart failure/venous congestion

Cardiac output is determined by a combination of stroke volume and heart rate. Blood volume, vascular capacity, venous return and myocardial contractility are some of the other factors.

HIGH CARDIAC OUTPUT

Causes
- Tachycardia < 160 b.p.m. (pyrexia, anxiety, exercise, carbon dioxide retention)
- Thyrotoxicosis

Problems
- Slow induction of anaesthesia when using volatile agents
- Possibility of high-output cardiac failure (heart failure is the inability to maintain an adequate cardiac output in a situation in which other cardiovascular variables are normal or where the other variables are so disturbed that the physiological limits on cardiac contraction are exceeded)

Assessment
- Clinical history and examination
- Central venous pressure
- Skin temperature

Preparation
Therapy should be started in an attempt to return the cardiac output to normal. Agents such as atropine that are likely to exacerbate the situation should be avoided.

FIXED CARDIAC OUTPUT

Causes
- Obstructive valvular heart disease
- Fixed heart rate
- Constrictive pericarditis
- Cardiac tamponade

Problems
The principal problem is an inability to withstand haemodynamic changes, e.g. in blood volume and low peripheral resistance. For example:
- Aortic stenosis—hypotension should be avoided as this increases the intraventricular pressure and thus reduces myocardial perfusion.
- Aortic incompetence—avoid hypertension to prevent rise in intraventricular pressure and reduction in myocardial perfusion.
- Mitral stenosis—a tachycardia leads to a reduction in ventricular filling and the cardiac output falls.
- Mitral incompetence—hypertension and bradycardia lead to an increase in regurgitation and thus a fall in cardiac output.

Assessment
- Clinical history and examination
- Chest X-ray (heart size, signs of left ventricular failure)
- ECG
- Specific investigations as necessary
  — Echocardiography
  — Cardiac catheterisation
  1. Preoperative preparation should achieve an optimal state for surgery
  2. Sedative premedication is used to minimise the adrenergic response to anxiety
  3. Preoxygenation should precede induction of anaesthesia
  4. When using intravenous induction agents take into account the altered circulation time. Administer the correct dose, at the correct speed, with close monitoring
  5. Maintenance of general anaesthesia—N_2O/O_2/neuromuscular blockade with or without analgesic plus IPPV
  6. Monitor ECG, blood pressure, pulse rate, S_pO_2 and ET_{CO_2}

AVOID
- Hypovolaemia
- Sudden vasodilatation
- Chronotropic agents (care with neostigmine and atropine, the use of glycopyrrolate preferable)
- Myocardial depressants such as inhalation agents especially halothane

Specific therapy for patients with valvular heart disease should include the use of prophylactic antibiotics to protect against sub-acute bacterial endocarditis.

LOW CARDIAC OUTPUT

1. Inadequate contractility
2. Inadequate preload
3. Excessive afterload
4. Inefficient heart rate: < 40 or > 160 b.p.m.

1. Inadequate contractility

Causes
- Ischaemic heart disease
- Cardiomyopathy
- Decompensated valvular heart disease

Problems
- Arrhythmias
- Low-output cardiac failure
- Ischaemic heart disease—stable angina, ST segment and T-wave changes have been found to be of minimal importance in

determining cardiac risk. A myocardial infarct within 6 months and rhythm disorders, however, are considered high risk factors.

- One-third of patients operated on within 3 months of an infarct reinfarct, and half of these die. During anaesthesia the heart-rate systolic-blood-pressure product should be kept below 16 000 (HR × BP = 80 × 120 = 9600); this is said to minimise cardiac work; hypotension, however, is undesirable, as coronary perfusion is compromised.
- Factors precipitating reinfarction are hypoxaemia, dehydration, increased metabolic demands, hypercoagulability and acute starvation.
- Ultimately the heart fails if its ability to contract continues to decline. Heart failure results in poor peripheral perfusion, reducing the efficiency of all organs.

Assessment
- Pulse, blood pressure
- Core/surface temperature difference
- Urine output
- Cerebral status

Preparation
- Treat heart failure if present
- Treat aggravating factors, e.g. obesity, hypertension
- Specific therapy as indicated

(See p. 21 for summary of the pathophysiology of myocardial oxygen flux.)

Management
1. Preoxygenation
2. Careful, gentle induction of anaesthesia (avoid relative overdose by careful attention to rate of injection)
3. Topical local anaesthetic to vocal cords and upper trachea (blood pressure, rise in heart rate and dysrhythmias reduced)
4. Routine monitoring

AVOID
- Hypoxia and hypercarbia
- Shivering (muscle oxygen demand ↑, cardiac output ↑, myocardial oxygen demand ↑, oxygen supply unchanged → **HYPOXAEMIA**)
- Agents likely to depress the myocardium without reducing the workload, e.g. beta blockers
- Excessive sympathetic activity
- 'Light anaesthesia'
- Rapid changes in blood volume

2. Inadequate preload

Causes
- Low blood volume
  — Renal failure (post-dialysis)
  — Inadequate fluid intake
  — Excessive fluid loss (vomiting, diarrhoea, haemorrhage)
- Phaeochromocytoma
- Massive vasodilatation
  — Gram negative septicaemia
  — Amniotic fluid embolism
- Vena caval obstruction
  — Supine hypotensive syndrome

An absolute hypovolaemia will lead to a low central venous pressure, as will a normal blood volume occupying a large vascular capacity, for example a massive peripheral vasodilation leading to blood stasis or pooling.

Problems
- Hypotension
- Poor perfusion

Assessment
- Heart rate, blood pressure, CVP, PCWP
- Core/surface temperature difference
- Urine output

Preparation
Treat with infusion of appropriate fluids to improve perfusion under close central venous pressure monitoring (Table 2.1).

Table 2.1 Relative merits of crystalloids, colloids, plasma and blood

Solution	Adverse reactions	Circulatory half-life (depending upon capillary integrity)
0.9% saline	−	
Haemaccel	+	30 min
Gelofusine	+	$1\frac{1}{2}$ h
Pentospan	+	hours
Dextran 70	+	$3\frac{1}{2}$ h
Plasma protein fraction	−	hours
Blood	+	days

Management
1. No premedication if peripheral perfusion poor (ventilatory and cardiovascular depression may result, leading to a further reduction in tissue oxygenation).

2. Ketamine/pancuronium technique: in the absence of maximal adrenergic drive both ketamine and pancuronium cause an increase in heart rate and blood pressure.
3. Infuse fluids to produce, or maintain, urine production.

AVOID
- A sudden fall in peripheral resistance or blood volume
- High intrathoracic pressures–reduces venous return

3. Excessive afterload

Caused by:
- Severe hypertension
- Severe coarctation

Management
Heart failure associated with hypertension is an indication for acute therapy. Frusemide and methyldopa are drugs of choice; hydralazine and prazosin, vasodilators are also effective in reducing the afterload. Other drugs that have been used are sodium nitroprusside, labetalol, diazoxide, clonidine and guanethidine.
   Coarctation may need urgent surgery if heart failure is present.

4. Inefficient heart rate (< 40 or > 160/min in the adult)

Causes of tachycardia
- Apprehension/anxiety ⎫
- Pyrexia   ⎪
- Pain   ⎬ Usually sinus rhythm
- Hypovolaemia   ⎪
- Hypercarbia   ⎭
- Ischaemic heart disease
  — Fast atrial fibrillation
  — Flutter
  — Ventricular tachycardia
- Endocrine disorders
  — Thyrotoxicosis
  — Phaeochromocytoma
- Pharmacologically induced
  — Parasympatholytic agents
  — Sympathomimetic agents

Causes of bradycardia
- Physiological sinus bradycardia
- Ischaemic heart disease
  — Heart block
- Pharmacologically induced
  — Digoxin
  — Beta adrenergic receptor blockade

Problems
Poor perfusion is the usual result, the tachycardia allows
insufficient time for adequate ventricular filling and a bradycardia
causes a fall in cardiac output because the stroke volume cannot
compensate for the low heart rate.

Management of common arrhythmias
- Sinus bradycardia: Atropine
- Sinus tachycardia: Beta adrenergic blockers
- Supraventricular arrhythmia: Beta blockers, verapamil,
                                  amiodarone
- Ventricular arrhythmia: Lignocaine, beta blockers,
                                  procainamide, quinidine,
                                  bretylium and amiodarone

Assessment
Assess state of poor perfusion as above.

Preparation
- Adjust dose of pharmacological agents if considered
  responsible, or change the drug
- Treat underlying pathology if possible
- Cardiac pacing may be necessary for:
  — Complete heart block
  — Stokes–Adams attacks

Management
- Minimise changes in blood volume and peripheral resistance by
  using appropriate agents in the correct dose and injection rate
  and adequate fluid replacement
- **CARE** with diathermy/pacing—check compatibility. An external
  pacing device should be available

Note: 'Demand' pacemakers are inhibited by impulses of frequency
within the normal physiological range.
    'Fixed-rate' pacemakers may trigger an R-on-T arrhythmia in
patients whose myocardium is irritable—this may occur during
anaesthesia (multiple ventricular ectopics, ventricular tachycardia
or ventricular fibrillation).
    Diathermy can totally inhibit a pacemaker, or turn a demand unit
into one of fixed rate. Use of diathermy within 15 cm of the
electrode or unit may destroy it.
1. The patient's heart rate should be monitored continuously
2. The indifferent diathermy pad should be as far away as possible
   from the pacemaker
3. A defibrillator and external pacing device should be at hand

AVOID
Agents likely to make the arrhythmia worse, e.g. atropine, glycopyrollate in patients with tachycardia, halothane or combinations of fentanyl and vecuronium in patients with bradycardia.

FAILURE OF OXYGENATION

Causes
- Right-to-left shunts (cyanotic congenital heart disease)
  — Fallot's tetralogy
  — Ebstein's anomaly
  — Tricuspid atresia
  — Transposition of great vessels
  — Pulmonary stenosis and atrial septal defect
  — Anomalous venous drainage
  — Eisenmenger's syndrome
- Pulmonary congestion
  — Mitral stenosis
  — Left ventricular failure

Problems
- Hypoxia (heart failure and arrhythmias)
- Pulmonary hypertension. This may occur naturally or may result from a Blalock procedure to improve oxygen saturation in the severely cyanosed patient. A systemic/pulmonary shunt is created. Pulmonary hypertension is common in longstanding mitral stenosis, VSD and left ventricular failure.

Assessment
- Clinical history and examination
- Exercise tolerance
- Cardiac catheterisation and angiography

Preparation
- Treat heart failure if present
- Control dysrhythmias
- Antibiotic cover to protect against sub-acute bacterial endocarditis

Management
1. Sedative premedication without ventilatory depression
2. Preoxygenation
3. ECG monitoring
4. Smooth, gentle induction of anaesthesia

AVOID
- Agents likely to change the haemodynamic state, such as ketamine which raises pulmonary artery pressure
- High intrathoracic pressures may reverse a left-to-right shunt, leading to cyanosis

DISORDERS OF VASOMOTOR CONTROL

An inability of the peripheral vasculature to respond to changes occuring elsewhere in the system renders the patient vulnerable.
1. Fixed tone
2. Variable tone
3. Chronic increased tone

1. Fixed tone
Cause—arteriosclerosis

General approach
• Myocardial depressants should be avoided, as should sudden changes in posture
• Electrocardiographic monitoring is essential
• Care should be taken to avoid trauma to the skin as healing may be impaired by the poor peripheral circulation

2. Variable tone
• Spinal lesion
• Autonomic neuropathy—diabetes, tetanus
• Phaeochromocytoma (p. 74)
• Carcinoid (p. 76)

General approach
Spinal cord lesions There may be an imbalance in vasomotor tone, though epidural local anaesthetic block has been used to improve the circulation in patients with poliomyelitis.
Autonomic reflexes may be obtunded and care should be taken to minimise the cardiovascular fluctuations that may occur.

Autonomic neuropathy Patients with longstanding diabetes may develop an autonomic neuropathy. This results in less fine control of the blood pressure and care should be taken during anaesthesia to avoid excess fluid loss as compensatory changes are less effective. There is an increased risk of acute cardiorespiratory death during and after surgery.

3. Chronic increased tone
Increase in arteriolar tone may result from a variety of conditions.

Essential hypertension
The aetiology of essential hypertension is thought to be due to a renal difficulty in excreting sodium. The blood volume would expand were it not for an increase in a circulating substance that inhibits sodium reabsorption in the tubules. A sodium transport inhibitor in the circulation, however, also affects other tissues; smooth muscle, being no exception, responds by an increase in tone. This increase in tone may become permanent.

Other conditions
- Reno-vascular disease (renal artery stenosis)
- Toxaemia of pregnancy
- Conn's syndrome

General management of the patient with hypertension
1. Control hypertension with beta-adrenergic receptor blockade and other anti-hypertensive agents
2. a. X-ray chest—heart size, left ventricular failure, aortic coarctation
   b. ECG—evidence of left ventricular failure and/or ischaemic heart disease
   c. Blood electrolytes
3. Normal premedication
4. Monitor CVP, BP, S_pO_2, F_ECO_2 and ECG
5. Preoxygenation
6. Neuroleptanaesthesia
   N_2O/O_2; Fentanyl/Droperidol; topical local anaesthetic to vocal cords and upper trachea
7. Endotracheal intubation
8. IPPV at normocapnia
9. No pressor agents
10. No myocardial depressants such as halothane

MYOCARDIAL O_2 CONSUMPTION

Oxygen consumption can be of several categories:
1. Basal O_2 demand
2. Heart rate $\uparrow$ ... consumption $\uparrow$
3. Contractility $\uparrow$ ... consumption $\uparrow$
4. Intraventricular pressure/size of ventricle varies with wall tension: tension $\uparrow$ ... consumption $\uparrow$. Thus if intraventricular pressure is raised then ... consumption $\uparrow$.

MYOCARDIAL O_2 SUPPLY

1. During diastole:
   The O_2 supply is proportional to blood flow, which is proportional to the coronary artery filling pressure/resistance multiplied by time.
   Diastolic time $\uparrow$ ... O_2 supply $\uparrow$
   Diastolic time $\downarrow$ ... O_2 supply $\downarrow$
   Thus, if the heart rate rises, oxygen delivery falls.
2. Local vasodilator metabolites $\rightarrow$ vasodilation $\rightarrow$ O_2 supply $\uparrow$
   AVOID hypertension ... intraventricular pressure $\uparrow$ .... O_2 supply $\downarrow$
   AVOID hypotension ... coronary artery filling pressure $\downarrow$ .... O_2 supply $\downarrow$
   AVOID tachycardia .... O_2 demand $\uparrow$ .... O_2 supply $\downarrow$
   AVOID hypoxia .... O_2 supply $\downarrow$

HAEMATOLOGICAL DISORDERS

Blood disorders have **FOUR** important functional components of interest to anaesthetists:
• Oxygen carriage
• Acute haemolysis of red cells
• Haemastasis
• Increased risk of thrombosis

OXYGEN CARRIAGE

Oxygen flux = Cardiac output $\times$ C_aO_2
$\qquad$ = $\dot{Q}_T \times [(S_aO_2 \times 1.34 \times Hb)$
$\qquad\qquad + (P_a \times$ sol. coeff. of O_2 in plasma)]
Oxygen consumption = Cardiac output $\times$ ($C_aO_2 - C_vO_2$)

1. The effects of cardiac output are dealt with under cardiovascular disturbances (p. 42).
2. The saturation of haemoglobin with oxygen is determined by many factors, many of them being of respiratory or cardiac/cardiovascular origin ($\dot{V}_a/\dot{Q}_c$ abnormalities or true shunts) and these are therefore dealt with in those sections (pp. 19, 39, 49).

Haemoglobin oxygen saturation is also determined by other factors. Factors affecting the affinity of the haemoglobin for oxygen:
• 2.3 DPG $\uparrow$ $\qquad\qquad$ Right shift
• pH [H]$^+$ $\uparrow$ $\qquad\qquad$ Right shift
• Temperature rise $\qquad\quad$ Right shift
• Haemoglobinopathies (p. 53)
• Carbon monoxide poisoning (p. 170)

3. Haemoglobin concentration is a major component of oxygen transport and there are many causes for abnormal haemoglobin levels.

Causes of anaemia
• Reduced erythropoiesis
 — Aplastic anaemia (various types)
 — Leukaemia
 — Renal disease
• Disordered cellular development
 — Vitamin B_{12} deficiency
 — Folic acid deficiency
• Reduced erythrocyte lifespan
 — Haemolysis
 — Autoimmune disease
 — Haemoglobinopathies
 — Drug-induced
 — Transfusion reaction
• Haemorrhage
• Plasma expansion

Management of the anaemic patient
A haemoglobin of about 11 g.dl^{-1} provides optimal oxygen delivery. Although the oxygen carrying capacity is reduced, total flow is increased and this results in a net increase in oxygen delivery.

If the haemoglobin concentration falls below 5 g.dl^{-1} hypoxaemia is difficult to detect.

Transfusion should normally be considered if the [Hb] is below 9–10 g.dl^{-1}; this should be carried out at least 24 h preoperatively to allow time for the regeneration of adequate levels of 2.3 DPG.

Causes of polycythaemia
• Chronic hypoxia
• Dehydration
• Polycythaemia vera

Management of the polycythaemic patient
A [Hb] of > 18 g.dl^{-1} is associated with a rise in blood viscosity such that the incidence of intravascular thrombosis is increased. Treated by venesection with appropriate colloid fluid replacement. The polycythaemic patient may appear cyanosed, even when oxygen carriage is adequate.

ACUTE HAEMOLYSIS OF RED CELLS

Transfusion reactions
Haemoglobinopathies
    Sickle cell syndromes:

Sickle cell trait	HbA + HbS (< 50%)
Sickle cell anaemia	HbS + HbS (90–95%) (5–10% HbF)
Sickle cell HbC disease	HbS + HbC (50:50)
Sickle cell thalassaemia	HbS + Thall

These conditions are inherited according to basic Mendelian laws.
    AS   ×   AS
AA   AS   AS   SS

HbS is most commonly found in central Africans (20% carrier rate), West Indians and in the northern USA (8% carrier rate). It is also found in Greece, in India and in the Middle East.

HbC is found commonly in northern Ghana—15%.

Beta thalassaemia is found around the Mediterranean, and in India, China and the Middle East.

'Sickling' depends on the amount of abnormal haemoglobin and the state of deoxygenation.

In general, SS and CC sickle at a Po_2 of 4–5 kPa (30–40 mmHg) and AS at 2.5 kPa (20 mmHg).

Problems
• Gelation of HbS ... sickling ... haemolytic crisis
• Anaemia

Preparation

Assessment
- Sickledex test (quick)
- Electrophoresis
- P_aO_2, S_pO_2
- Preoperative transfusion if Hb < 5 g.dl^{-1}
- Exchange transfusion in cases of very major surgery
- Treatment of infection if present

Management
- Avoid hypoxia during and after anaesthesia
- Monitor oxygen saturation
- Avoidance of circulatory stasis, hypothermia and acidosis
- The administration of alkalis has been suggested by some
- Use simple, familiar techniques
- Avoid tourniquets if possible

HAEMOSTASIS

The most common diseases are those of haemophilia, thrombocytopaenia, hypofibrinogenaemia, post-transfusion coagulopathy and anticoagulant therapy.

Haemophilia
- Coagulation disorders 90% due to haemophilia. Factor VIII must be replaced prior to surgery; use cryoprecipitate 20–30 ml per bag.
- 2 units/12 kg body weight is given initially.
- 1 unit/12 kg body weight is given 12-hourly for maintenance.
- The biological half-life of Factor VIII is 12 h.

Thrombocytopaenia
When transfusion is indicated, blood that is less than 12 h old or platelet concentrates should be given. Retinal haemorrhages are considered a positive indication for transfusion; however, if a splenectomy is proposed, give the transfusion after excision of the spleen.

Hypofibrinogenaemia
This may be the result of disseminated intravascular coagulation (DIC). A full clotting 'screen' is important because DIC is a dynamic process and treatment changes depend on the actual state of the process.

The critical fibrinogen level is 100 mg.dl^{-1}. A platelet count and the assessment of fibrin degradation products (FDP) may clarify the situation. Excessive coagulation causes a thrombocytopaenia; excessive fibrinolysis increases the FDP.

Post-transfusion coagulopathy
1. Platelet deficiency
2. Factor V absent in ACD blood
3. Dilution of the patient's own coagulation factors

Management
- Clotting 'screen'
- Platelets, fresh frozen plasma
- Fresh blood

Anticoagulant therapy
The prothrombin time should be maintained 1.5–2.5 times the control value. Vitamin K should only be used if absolutely necessary as its effect on anticoagulation may be prolonged.

INCREASED RISK OF THROMBOSIS

Five variables have been shown to identify patients at risk: euglobulin lysis time, serum concentration of fibrin-related antigen, age, excess weight and varicose veins. Other preoperative factors have also been associated with a higher risk of thrombosis. These include cigarette smoking, polycythaemia and the contraceptive pill.

The type of surgery, gynaecological in particular, and postoperative immobility have also been included in the list of factors predisposing to deep vein thrombosis and pulmonary embolism.

Management
- Lose excess weight
- Stop smoking
- Stop taking the contraceptive pill for at least 3 months (the risk of thrombosis has to be set against the risk of pregnancy)
- Use of devices which enhance venous blood flow in the legs (inflatable boots, mechanical flexion/extension of the foot)
- Early ambulation
- The use of prophylactic subcutaneous heparin or low molecular weight heparin has to be weighed against the associated increased risk of bleeding
- It is likely that the use of a predictive index of risk, and to treat only those at risk, is the future ideal solution

RENAL DISEASE

There are **TWO** main aspects of acute renal disease; they are:
1. Failure of correct osmole excretion
2. Failure of correct water excretion
These may co-exist.

1. Incorrect osmole excretion $\begin{cases} \text{too much — nephrotic syndrome} \\ \text{too little — renal tubular dysfunction} \end{cases}$

2. Incorrect water excretion $\begin{cases} \text{too much —} \begin{cases} \text{high-output renal failure} \\ \text{diabetes insipidus} \end{cases} \\ \text{too little — low-output failure} \end{cases}$

Problems

The problems associated with renal disease can be divided into three groups: pathophysiological, infective and pharmacokinetic.

PATHOPHYSIOLOGICAL

1. Anaemia (p. 52)
The anaemia secondary to renal disease is thought to be partially due to a disordered haemopoietin secretion.

2. Acidosis/electrolyte imbalance (p. 58)
Both acidosis and electrolyte imbalance result from the kidneys' inability to control the passive or active absorption of ions from the tubules. Acid/base control is taken over by the lungs.

3. Arrhythmias (p. 47)
The dysrhythmias associated with renal disease are those that are normally associated with potassium disturbances.

4. Abnormal blood volume (p. 58)
Untreated renal failure leads to an increase in blood volume whereas the recently dialysed patient may be severly hypovolaemic.

INFECTIVE

Patients with renal failure are particularly susceptible to hepatitis B infection, especially those that have undergone haemodialysis. It is not routine to screen for the hepatitis B surface antigen (HBsAG) but it should be considered in those patients who are at risk and precautions should be taken; if found to be positive, gown-up, wear surgical gloves, wear goggles and incinerate all material contaminated with blood or body fluids.

PHARMACOKINETIC

Tissue affinity for drugs may be altered and their binding to plasma proteins changed. To induce sleep in the patient with renal failure a smaller dose of thiopentone is required than in the normal patient. Only infrequently does hypoproteinaemia increase the unbound active form of the drug.

Prolonged apnoea following suxamethonium is often associated with haemodialysis—there is a relative lack of pseudocholinesterase. If more than 50% of a drug is excreted through the kidneys then dosage adjustment is necessary according to the glomerular filtration rate.

An ideal drug in renal failure should
- not be nephrotoxic
- be < 30% excreted through the kidney
- have no active metabolites
- be unaffected by protein levels

Assessment
- Clinical history and examination
- Full blood count
- Urea and electrolytes
- Australia antigen
- Plasma proteins

Preparation
- Consider transfusion
- There is still debate about the wisdom of preoperative transfusion in the patient with chronic renal failure as immunological and haematological problems may result
- Identify acceptable electrolyte limits

For the patient on regular dialysis electrolyte control should be good; less ideal values may have to be accepted in those in urgent need of surgery and not on dialysis.

MANAGEMENT OF THE PATIENT WITH RENAL DISEASE

The management of the renal patient has two aims:
- To perform anaesthesia successfully with the physiological and pharmacological problems described above
- To avoid causing further derangement to impaired renal function

1. Renal blood flow must be maintained
Anaesthesia abolishes autoregulation. Thus if the blood pressure falls below 80 mmHg renal blood flow (RBF) will fall, glomerular filtration decreases and urine output drops.
a. inhalation agents ...... RBF $\downarrow$ 40%—depends on the agent and the arterial pressure fall is proportional to the dose
b. Thiopentone/N_2O relaxant ...... RBF $\downarrow$ 30%
c. Spinal anaesthesia .... RBF $\downarrow$ proportional to fall in arterial pressure
2. Antidiuretic hormone secretion should be minimised
a. Barbiturates .... ADH secretion does not increase
b. Narcotics .... ADH secretion does not increase
   (High-dose narcotic analgesics impair the ADH response to stress)
c. Phenothiazines .... ADH secretion falls

AVOID
Fluorinated ethers
Fluorine concentrations rise following biotransformation of the agent, and these levels may be increased if the agent is given in

high concentrations for a prolonged period of time or if enzyme induction has occurred.

The result of excess free fluorine ions is to produce an ADH-resistant polyuria which then becomes an oliguria; urea and potassium ultimately rise.

ASSESSMENT OF FLUID AND ELECTROLYTE BALANCE

Extra-cellular fluid volume (ECF)

Decrease: Loss of fluid into the intestinal tract
Renal losses
Burns
Osmotic diuresis
Addison's disease
Phaeochromocytoma

Increase: Excessive administration of fluids
Renal failure
Congestive cardiac failure
Hepatic cirrhosis
Cushing's disease

Assessment: Clinical history
BP, heart rate, pulse volume
Fullness of veins
Central venous pressure, oedema
Urinary output/fluid balance
Chest X-ray

Treatment: Treat causal process
Fluid administration must depend upon the fluid balance and upon the result of the dynamic testing of the central venous pressure

Tonicity

Decrease: Excess water load (5% dextrose)
Congestive cardiac failure
K^+ depletion (Na^+ replaces intracellular K^+)
Excess ADH production
Liver disease

Increase: Excessive losses, e.g. diabetes insipidus
Inadequate water intake

Assessment: Clinical history and examination
Electrolyte changes are small initially in states of water intoxication, decreased tonicity, but later the $[Na^+]$ falls to < 135 mmol.l^{-1}—give 5% dextrose
Blood volume is well maintained initially in states of dehydration, increased tonicity but later the [Hb] and PCV rise, and urine output falls—give 5% dextrose

Potassium concentration

Decrease: Vomiting, diarrhoea

Diuretics
Steroid therapy (Cushing's disease)
Diuretic phase of renal failure
Renal tubular acidosis
Villous papilloma
Aldosteronism (Conn's syndrome)

Assessment: Urea and electrolytes
Fluid balance
Treatment: Check that the urine output is satisfactory, then administer parenteral potassium < 20 mmol.h^{-1} or < 200 mmol.day^{-1}
Increase: Failure of excretion
Acidosis
Spironolactone
Addison's disease
Assessment: Clinical history
Urea and electrolytes
Creatinine
pH
fluid balance
Treatment: Glucose 50 g
Soluble insulin 24 units
100 ml NaHCO$_3$ 8.4%
10% calcium gluconate 10 ml
Resonium A
Peritoneal dialysis
Haemodialysis

(A urinary [Na$^+$] > 30 mmol.l^{-1} and a urinary urea concentration of > 1.1 g.dl^{-1} is suggestive of intrinsic renal failure.)

LIVER DYSFUNCTION

There are **four** functional aspects to liver dysfunction that are of interest to the anaesthetist:
1. Jaundice
2. Increased risk of bleeding
   a. Failure of coagulation
   b. Portal hypertension
3. Failure of detoxication
4. Australia antigen (hepatitis B surface antigen [HBsAg])

Increased haemoglobin degradation } $\rightarrow$ Jaundice
Obstructive liver disease   } $\rightarrow$
          ↓   ↓
Hepatocellular disease → { Coagulation defects
                          Reduced detoxication
                          Portal hypertension
                          Australia antigen [HBsAg]

JAUNDICE

Causes
- Increased haemoglobin degradation
  — Haemolysis
  — Resorption of haematoma
- Obstructive liver disease
  — Cholelithiasis
  — Cholestasis
  — Cancer of the head of pancreas
- Hepatocellular disease
  — Hepatitis
  — Cirrhosis
  — Poisoning

HAEMORRHAGE

- Coagulation defects—reduced production of coagulation proteins
- Oesophageal varices—may rupture spontaneously, or as a result of trauma, nasogastric intubation

FAILURE OF DETOXICATION

- Choice of drugs and dosages difficult
- The effect of a drug in hepatic diseases is not very predictable as there is considerable overlap between doses required for the patient with liver disease and for the normal population

RISK OF HEPATITIS B

Take precaution if HBsAg positive (p. 122)

MANAGEMENT OF THE PATIENT WITH LIVER DISEASE:

Assessment
- Clinical history and examination
- Drug history
- Liver function tests
- Plasma proteins
- Serum urea and electrolytes
- Coagulation 'screen'
- Blood ammonia
- Australia antigen 'screen'

Preparation
- Vitamin K therapy if abnormal prothrombin time
- Platelets if required
- Transfusion if anaemic

- Pre-induction infusion of mannitol (bladder catheterisation)
- Precautions against AA (HBsAg) contamination

The anaesthetic management of the patient with liver disease should be such that further liver dysfunction is minimised.

1. Premedication
Care should be taken with opiates: halve the dose, as excretion may be halved. Benzodiazepines differ in their pharmokinetic profiles—oxazepam excretion is unchanged; however, the dose of diazepam should be reduced.

2. Induction
If the patient has obstructive jaundice a mannitol infusion should be given. It is thought that in obstructive jaundice toxins are absorbed from the gut, and not removed by the liver, and it is the concentration of these toxins in the kidney that may be the causative agent in the renal failure that is termed 'the hepato-renal syndrome'. Diuretics, by increasing tubular flow, dilute these toxins. Catheterisation is necessary. The patients most at risk are those with bilirubin concentrations of > 140 µmol.l^{-1}. (In addition, diuretics protect the kidney from hypoxic damage, as they reduce the metabolic work that the tubular cells perform.)

Intravenous barbiturates are satisfactory for the induction of anaesthesia but they may accumulate if repeated doses are given. The dose of suxamethonium required may be less because of the lower levels of pseudocholinesterase.

3. Care with nasogastric tubes if oesophageal varices are suspected
Maintenance: The dose of non-depolarising drugs may need to be large to produce effective relaxation. Liver dysfunction does not affect the duration of action of inhalational agents as elimination is predominantly via the lungs.

AVOID
- Agents that are predominantly broken down in the liver
- Prolonged fasting—as the glycogen-depleted liver is at greater risk from the toxic effects of the pharmacological agents
- Hypotension—poor perfusion leading to hypoxia enhances the toxicity of other agents
- Enxyme induction—increased metabolism of drugs leads to an increase in the concentration of toxic free radicals
- Known hepatoxic agents

Jaundice following general anaesthesia and surgery
There is some epidemiological evidence to suggest that multiple anaesthetics/operations over a relatively short period increase the incidence of postoperative jaundice. Halothane has been implicated as a causal agent.

Hypotension, hypoxaemia and hypercarbia can all lead to liver dysfunction and therefore these side-effects should be minimised in all general anaesthetic procedures. It is likely that a combination of circumstances, perhaps anaerobic reductive biodegradation of halothane and the combination of the resultant metabolites with protein, may provoke liver failure in a patient with a genetic 'immunological' predisposition. The entity of 'halothane hepatitis' is rare.

When it is necessary to give multiple anaesthetics over a short period (3-monthly intervals) it is wise to administer an agent other than halothane from a 'halothane-free' anaesthetic machine.

DISORDERS OF THE BRAIN, SPINAL CORD, NERVES AND MUSCLE

CENTRAL NERVOUS SYSTEM

Disorders of the central nervous system can be divided into two groups:
1. Where the cooperation of the patient is limited by an intellectual or psychological defect:
   a. Mental retardation/dementia/confusion
   b. Psychiatric disorders
2. Where there is an intracranial disease process that requires special management:
   a. Epilepsy
   b. Raised intracranial pressure
   c. Cerebral aneurysm
   d. Parkinsonism
   e. Deranged blood/brain barrier

Mental retardation/dementia/confusion

Causes
Many idiopathic syndromes:
- Cerebral dysfunction due to
  — Hypoxia
  — Hypoglycaemia
  — Hypercarbia
  — Uraemia
  — Hepatic failure, etc.
- Cerebral damage due to
  — Head injury
  — Infection
- Inborn errors of metabolism

Problems
- Possible lack of cooperation

- Concomitant pathology associated with many of the conditions:
  — Congenital heart disease
  — Endocrine disturbance

Management
1. Parenteral premedication should be avoided in the uncooperative patient. An oral tranquilliser is appropriate and profound sedation may be desirable in the grossly disturbed patient.
2. Patients with an organic confusional state are not improved by the administration of drugs; however, drugs that are completely metabolished or eliminated quickly are the least likely to cause problems.

Psyhiatric disorders
Most anaesthetic-related problems are associated with drug therapy (p. 30)
- Tricyclic antidepressants
- Monoamine oxidase inhibitors
- Lithium

Epilepsy

Causes
- Idiopathic
- Cerebral trauma or surgery
- Tumours
- Drug therapy

Problems
- Induction of enzymes by phenobarbitone, and to a lesser extent by phenytoin, may increase the toxicity of other drugs.
- Competition for degradation pathways may increase the concentration of circulating drugs, such as phenytoin, by diazepam.

Management
It is important to know the frequency of attacks. Specific drug therapy, phenytoin, sodium valproate, diazepam (for grand mal), and ethosuximide (for petit mal).

Premedication
- Use drugs with anticonvulsant action—diazepam.
- Induction and maintenance of anaesthesia with drugs with inherent anticonvulsant properties e.g. thiopentone.
- Avoid drugs likely to increase the excitability of the cerebral cortex (ketamine, methoxyflurane, enflurane). Isoflurane also has been associated with convulsions.
- There is some evidence that patients taking phenytoin have increased sensitivity to non-depolarising agents.

Raised intracranial pressure (ICP)

Causes
- Trauma/oedema
- Tumour
- Hydrocephalus

Assessment
- Clinical history and examination
- Optic fundi—papilloedema
- Intracranial pressure monitoring (p. 150)

Preparation

Steroids ⎫
Fluid restriction ⎬ Reduces oedema and therefore reduces pressure
Osmotic diuretics ⎭

Ventricular drainage   Removes CSF—reduces pressure

Management

Avoid depressant premedication ⎫ P_aCO_2 normal or low
No coughing or straining ⎪   Venous pressure minimal
Perfect airway (armoured tube) ⎬   Cerebral perfusion pressure
Adequate ventilation (IPPV) ⎪   lowered
Minimal expiratory resistance ⎪   ↓
Blood pressure not elevated ⎭

Reduces cerebral blood volume
↓
Reduces intracranial pressure

P_aCO_2 < 2.5 kPa (20 mmHg) leads to cerebral vasoconstriction—hypoxia. A mean BP < 60 mmHg reduces cerebral blood flow such that ischaemia may occur.

Minimal concentrations of volatile anaesthetic agents are used—high concentrations cause cerebral vasodilation and thus increase intracranial blood volume and hence intracranial pressure.

Cerebral aneurysm

Problems

'Steal' and 'inverse steal'

Damaged brain vasculature does not respond to metabolites in the same way as intact brain. If the P_aCO_2 is raised the normal brain vasculature dilates and 'steals' blood flow from the damaged area. Conversely, hypocapnia leads to vasoconstriction of the normal vasculature and the damaged area is preferentially perfused. Avoid extremes. A bleed from an aneurysm leads to spasm and an area of cerebral ischaemia. Hypotension should be avoided as this may aggravate the hypoxia. Hypertension should be avoided as a further bleed may result. The intracranial pressure should be maintained so that the aneurysm is not unsupported. A smooth anaesthetic with cardiovascular stability is required.

Assessment
- Clinical presentation
- Computerised axial tomography CT scan
- Carotid angiography

Parkinsonism

Problems
Spasticity occurs, leading to limitation of mobility.

Management
The management of patients with Parkinson's disease requires the reduction of the spasticity by drug therapy—levodopa; this facilitates mobility and clearing of chest secretions by allowing greater activity.

Deranged blood/brain barrier
- Meningitis/encephalitis
- Multiple sclerosis

Problems
Drugs pass to the brain in concentrations that are toxic, e.g. local anaesthetic concentration threshold for convulsions is lowered.

Management of the patient with multiple sclerosis
Assessment: Note the natural history of the patient's disease
Enquire if the patient suffers from epilepsy: there is an increased incidence
Respiratory function tests
Preparation: Any infection should be treated vigorously as pyrexia is associated with relapse
Subcutaneous heparin should be given as there is increased platelet 'stickiness'
Anaesthesia: **AVOID** atropine—it may cause a rise in temperature
Diazepam premedication is safe
AVOID suxamethonium—[K^+] may rise and cause arrhythmias
Non-depolarising muscle relaxants should be used with caution: use a low dose
Consider prophylactic use of anti-pyretics
LA and spinal techniques are best avoided

DISORDERS OF THE SPINAL CORD AND PERIPHERAL NERVES

Anaesthetic-orientated problems associated with diseases of the spinal cord and peripheral nerves are of three types—cardiovascular stability, potassium release associated with the use of suxamethonium, and respiratory inadequacy.

Cardiovascular stability
- Poliomyelitis—unstable
- Multiple sclerosis—unstable
- Traumatic cord transection—unstable

Stability of serum potassium levels following the use of suxamethonium
- Poliomyelitis—stable
- Multiple sclerosis—unstable
- Traumatic cord transection—unstable
- Polyneuropathy—unstable

Respiratory involvement
Adequacy of ventilation depends on the level at which cord damage has occurred and which peripheral nerves are involved.

NEUROMUSCULAR DISORDERS

The functional importance of the neuromuscular disorders can be described by their effect on muscle power, and thus on ventilatory ability, and also the response to the various drugs used to block the neuromuscular junction or alter muscle tone.

Respiratory inadequacy (p. 41)

Abnormal response to neuromuscular blocking agents

1. Depolarising agents (suxamethonium)

Atypical cholinesterase	— extended duration of blockade
Myasthenia gravis	— recovery occurs within minutes but may be incomplete
Myasthenic syndrome	— extremely sensitive
Dystrophia myotonia	— myotonia increased
Progressive muscular dystrophy	— a small dose should be given and its effect noted

2. Non-depolarising agents

Myasthenia gravis	— extreme sensitivity
Myasthenic syndrome	— extreme sensitivity
Dystrophia myotonia	— neuromuscular transmission is blocked but myotonia may persist
Progressive muscular dystrophy	— a small dose should be given and the effect noted

Atypical cholinesterase
Enzymatic hydrolysis is the chief factor controlling the plasma level of suxamethonium—, less than 5% of the injected dose reaches the neuromuscular junction. Of the population 96.2% are the 'normal' heterozygote and they hydrolyse suxamethonium rapidly, whereas 3.8% are heterozygote and hydrolysis takes 5–10 minutes. One in 2800 is the atypical homozygote and hydrolysis is prolonged.

There are Dibucaine and fluoride 'resistant' genes and a silent gene. Prolonged apnoea should be managed by mechanical ventilation with sedation until the spontaneous recovery occurs. The use of anticholinesterase in the final stages of recovery, or purified enzyme, is not standard practice.

Myasthenia gravis
Autoimmune reduced sensitivity to acetylcholine.
Assessment: Response to anticholinesterase
Pulmonary function tests/chest X-ray
Preparation: Anticholinesterase treatment is stopped preoperatively if the patient is able to manage—this reduces bronchorrhoea and produces a partial neuromuscular block. Depressant drugs are best avoided.
Anaesthesia: Induction with minimal thiopentone, or propofol N_2O, O_2 and halothane usually allows intubation, and adequate relaxation. Atracurium is the ideal muscle relaxant for these patients. Reversal of relaxation is not usually necessary.

APUD CELL DISORDERS (Endocrine and neuro-transmitter disorders)

APUD cells are of neuroectoderm origin and secrete amines and peptides; they are found in the pituitary, pancreas, adrenal glands, thyroid, parathyroids and in carcinoid tumours.

1. Abnormal glucocorticoid levels $\begin{cases} \text{Excessively high} \\ \text{Potentially inadequate} \end{cases}$

2. Abnormal glucose level $\begin{cases} \text{Low ketotic} \\ \text{High non-ketotic} \end{cases}$

3. Inappropriate metabolic rate $\begin{cases} \text{High} \\ \text{Low} \end{cases}$

4. Failure of calcium homeostasis $\begin{cases} \text{High calcium} \\ \text{Low calcium} \end{cases}$

5. Abnormal vasoactive 'hormones/transmitters' $\begin{cases} \text{Catecholamines} \\ \text{Kinins} \end{cases}$

Excessively high glucocorticoid levels

Causes
• High-dose steroid therapy
• Cushing's disease

Problems
- Fluid retention (p. 58)
- Potassium depletion (p. 58)
- Hypernatraemia
- Hypertension (p. 50)
- Impaired glucose tolerance (p. 70)
- Reduced protein synthesis (poor healing)
- Osteoporosis
- Muscle weakness

Assessment
Adrenal function tests:
- Plasma cortisol
- ACTH or Tetracosactrin response
- Response to insulin-induced hypoglycaemia (tests afferent and efferent pathways)
- Metapyrone test (tests efferent pathway)

Preparation
Treat hypertension, electrolyte imbalance and glucose intolerance.

Management
Glucocorticoid supplementation is essential, and in greater doses than normally used (200 mg hydrocortisone 6-hourly), because of the adaptation of tissues to very high levels. Weaning from steroids should be carried out slowly.

Potentially inadequate glucocorticoid levels

Causes
- Suppression of adrenal cortex due to steroid therapy
- Bilateral adrenalectomy
- Addison's disease
- Autoimmune adrenalitis (80% of cases)
- Tuberculosis
- Adrenal haemorrhage, infarction
- Meningococcal septicaemia
- Amyloidosis
- Hypopituitarism
- Trauma
- Infection
- Space-occupying lesion

Problems
- Hypertension
- Inability to respond to stressful situations—impaired reflex circulatory control—hypotension, 'shock'
- Weakness
- Possible sensitivity to narcotics

Assessment
Adrenal function tests:
• Pituitary/adrenal axis function tests as above
• High plasma ACTH, low cortisol—primary adrenocortical insufficiency
• Check adequacy of other endocrine systems

Preparation
• Addison's disease—replacement therapy for all zones of the cortex
• Secondary adrenal insufficiency—glucocorticoid replacement only
  — Glucocorticoid: Cortisol 20 mg 0800 h
                                  10 mg 1800 h
  — Mineralocorticoid: Fludrocortisone 0.05–0.15 mg daily

Management
Additional steriod cover is required during surgery, hydrocortisone (100 mg 6-hourly). There is an increased sensitivity to narcotics and barbiturates. The benzodiazepines are recommended for premedication.

Low glucose level

Causes
• Antidiabetic medication in excess of needs
  — Insulin-treated diabetics and those on chlorpropramide at risk
• Post-alcohol hypoglycaemia
• Insulinoma

Problems
Severe hypoglycaemia leads to brain damage.

Assessment
• Fasting blood sugar
• Glucose tolerance test
• Urinalysis—risk if always free of sugar

Preparation
Check control of diabetes:
• If controlled with insulin:
  — Stabilise on short-acting preparation if using a long-acting agent
  — Perform fasting blood sugar on day of operation
  — Set up an insulin and dextrose infusion to replace usual calorie intake prior to theatre
  — Arrange operation for the earliest time—less important for the patient who is well controlled
• If taking oral hypoglycaemic agents:
  — Stop 24 h preoperatively

Management
Regularly monitor blood sugar using a stick test or meter.

AVOID
- Discontinuation of calorie intake whilst maintaining insulin treatment
- Heavy premedication or anaesthesia—the patient's state of consciousness should be assessed at the end of the procedure Check blood sugar at end of surgery.

High glucose levels

Causes
- Untreated or inadequately treated diabetes mellitus
- Insulin resistance (found in sick patients)
- Insulin antagonism (excess growth hormone)

Problems
- Acidosis
- Hypokalaemia (p. 58)

Assessment
- Blood sugar
- Urea and electrolytes
- Investigate reason for lack of diabetic control (infection, other endocrine abnormalities)

Preparation
Delay surgery if possible so that the diabetic state can be controlled.
   Uncontrolled diabetes is a contraindication to anaesthesia/surgery except when immediate surgery is indicated or when drainage of an abcess is essential for the management of the diabetes and thus anaesthesia is necessary. Ketoacidosis should be controlled with a regime of dextrose/insulin/potassium with close biochemical and clinical monitoring. Extremely urgent surgery, which cannot be delayed, associated with ketoacidosis and hyperkalaemia has a high mortality.

Management
- Dextrose/insulin/potassium infusion with biochemical control, monitor intra-operative blood sugar
- ECG monitoring
- Take precaution to prevent pulmonary aspiration: diabetics are at great risk
- Use a balanced anaesthestic technique

AVOID
Underventilation

High metabolic rate

Causes
- Pyrexia
- Thyrotoxicosis—excessive production of T3/T4
  Problems associated with thyrotoxicosis:
  — Enlarged thyroid—possible upper airway compression (p. 91)
  — High cardiac output (p. 43)
  — Excessive adrenergic activity (p. 47), tachycardia, dysrhythmias—atrial fibrillation common
  — Myopathy
  — Possible thyrotoxic crisis

Assessment
- Clinical history and examination
- Isotope uptake (^{99}Tc, ^{131}I, ^{132}I)
- T3 and T4 levels
- Protein-bound iodine
- ECG
- X-ray of thoracic inlet—to identify tracheal patency

Preparation
- Specific therapy
- Antithyroid medication where indicated (including beta blockers)
- Antibiotics/antipyretics/active cooling

Management
Specific therapy:
- Pyrexia — antipyretics, antibiotics if indicated, active cooling
- Thyrotoxicosis — 1. Carbimazole } Blocks binding of iodine to
                      Methimazole } mono- and di-iodotyrosine
                      Thiouracils
                   2. Radioactive iodine (patients over 40 years)
                   3. Beta-adrenergic receptor blockade

   If possible, avoid atropine, which reduces sweating and therefore heat loss is decreased. Premedication with phenothiazines is reported to enhance anti-thyroid drugs and reduce thyrotrophin secretion. General anaesthesia is normally well tolerated in the absence of heart failure; ECG monitoring, however, is essential. An acute surgical emergency may precipitate a state of severe and uncontrolled thyrotoxicosis which is termed a 'thyrotoxic crisis'.
a. Hyperpyrexia
b. Confusion, restlessness, delirium, apathy, prostration
c. Tachycardia, atrial fibrillation, cardiac failure
d. Flushing and sweating
e. Vomiting, diarrhoea and abdominal pain
f. Dehydration and ketosis

Treatment
- Oxygen
- Sedation
- Fluid and electrolyte replacement
- Surface cooling
- Sodium iodide (0.5 g i.v. every 4 h)
- Carbimazole—for later benefit
- Beta-adrenergic blockade
- Hydrocortisone, should adrenal failure occur
- Nitroprusside for hypertension
- Digitalis for congestive heart failure

Low metabolic rate

Causes
- Hypothermia
- Myxoedema

Problems
- Low cardiac output, low heart rate, poor contractility—myocardial ischaemia (p. 44)
- Poor ability to metabolise drugs—therefore dose may need to be reduced.
- Possible pituitary/adrenal hypofunction (p. 68)
- Possible polyneuropathy

Assessment
- Clinical history and examination
- Temperature
- ECG
- Serum electrolytes and blood sugar (inappropriate ADH secretion)
- Clotting 'screen'
- Thyroid function tests (as above)

Preparation
Anaesthesia in the presence of severe myxoedema is associated with a high mortality. Postpone surgery if possible. Hypothermia may protect the patient against acute hypoxia but care is needed to avoid further depression of cardiac function.

The myxoedematous patient should be treated with triiodothyronine (peak effect 48–72 h) in an attempt to return physiological function to normal, although this may lead to dysrhythmia and heart failure. The ECG must be monitored.

Hydrocortisone is necessary to protect the patient against adrenocortical insufficiency. The hypothermic patient should be allowed to regain normal temperature if there is no need for hypothermia. Passive warming techniques are preferable to active 'surface' techniques (see below); these avoid the danger of burning the patient's skin.

Management
1. Premedication–usually avoided.
2. Use very small doses of drugs and assess their effect with care
3. Maintain the blood volume carefully
4. Monitor the ECG
5. Core and surface temperature (consider active 'central' rewarming if core temperature below 30°C)
6. Adjust ventilation to maintain a normal P_aco_2 (CO_2 solubility ↑ as temperature ↓)

AVOID
- Overventilation
- Large changes in haemodynamic performance
- Large surface/core temperature gradient—may lead to profound changes in core temperature if the patient's limbs are moved or elevated, and this may result in ventricular fibrillation
- Damage to skin: if a heated blanket is used then the blanket temperature should be only 1–2°C above the patient's surface temperature
- Chronotropic drugs

Note
Infection is common and congestive cardiac failure is easily precipitated. Myxoedema coma has a mortality of 80% and can be caused by carbon dioxide retention.

High calcium levels

Causes
- Hyperparathyroidism
  — Primary—adenoma, hyperplasia, carcinoma
  — Secondary to renal failure

Problems
- Muscle weakness (sensitivity to muscle relaxant)
- Spontaneous fractures
- Restricted thoracic cavity

Assessment
- Clinical history and examination
- Serum calcium level (raised)
- Chest X-ray, skeletal survey
- ECG
- Urea and electrolytes
- Radioimmunoassay of parathormone
- Electromyography
- Pulmonary function tests

Preparation
• Calcitonin

Management
• Anaesthesia is not normally associated with problems related to abnormal calcium levels alone.
• Use relaxants cautiously (use nerve stimulator to assess the degree and nature of block).
• Take care when moving and posturing the patient—the skeleton may be fragile.
• Control breathing if respiratory function is poor.

Low calcium levels

Causes
• Hypoparathyroidism (1% of patients post-thyroidectomy)
• Excess citrate (stored blood)
• Post-parathyroidectomy for hyperparathyroidism

Problem
If calcium ion concentration < 1.25 mmol—tetany
— laryngeal spasm
— cardiac irritability

Assessment
• Clinical history and examination (possible tetany)
• Serum calcium concentration low
• Urea and electrolytes
• Plasma proteins
• Electromyography

Preparation
• Parathyroid hormone
• Calcium
• Vitamin D

Management
1. Treat hypocalcaemia
2. Use relaxants with care (use nerve stimulator to assess degree and type of block)
3. Monitor ECG
4. Consider additional calcium during massive transfusions

AVOID
• Hyperventilation—alkalosis decreases ionised calcium
• Excess infusion of alkaline fluids

Phaeochromocytoma
A chromaffin tissue tumour: hypertension occurs in 90% of cases, it is paroxysmal in 40%.

Problems
- Sympathetic overactivity
- Diminished blood volume
- Possible hyperglycaemia

Assessment
- Clinical history and examination
- ECG
- Hb or PCV—high values indicate a low blood volume
- Metanephrine excretion (> 1.3 mg/24 h)
- Imaging techniques and selective sampling from inferior vena cava to determine tumour sites
- Blood sugar

Preparation
- Alpha-adrenergic receptor blockade (10–14 days) with phenoxybenzamine orally
- Gradual restoration of blood volume
- Beta-adrenergic receptor blockade provides background antiarrhythmia cover

Anaesthesia
Sedative premedication
Routine monitoring with intra-arterial pressure, CVP
Hypertension is controlled by intermittent phentolamine (1–5 mg i.v.) or by sodium nitroprusside (SNP) infusion. The systolic blood pressure should be maintained at about 80 mmHg.

The total dose of SNP should not exceed 0.5 $mg.kg^{-1}$ and the infusion rate should not exceed 0.01 $mg.kg^{-1}.min^{-1}$.

High dosage overloads the metabolic pathway and free cyanide is formed. Metabolic acidosis occurs as anaerobic metabolism predominates.

Treat hypotension with fluid infusion; if this is ineffective a pressor agent may be necessary: methoxamine, or metaraminol—but use with care.

A neuroleptanaesthesia technique with IPPV is suitable.

AVOID
- Hypoxia, hypercarbia, histamine release, sympathetic agents, handling the tumour, fear, stress and pain
- Halothane—because of its potential for cardiac dysrhythmias in the presence of adrenaline
- Suxamethonium—fasciculations may cause compression of the tumour, releasing catecholamine

Postoperative morbidity is often due to unresponsive hypo- or hypertension, leading to congestive heart failure or a cerebrovascular accident.

Carcinoid

This was originally called 'carcinoid' because it ran a more benign course than other carcinomas.

The secretion of kallikrein (which catalyses the conversion of kininogen to bradykinin) and 5-hydroxytryptamine (5HT) causes flushing, diarrhoea and bronchospasm in a small proportion of patients with the tumour. Triscupsid and pulmonary stenosis may also occur. 5HT and bradykinin cannot be detoxified in the liver when these are secreted by a metastasis distal to the liver; this leads to symptoms.

Problems
- Possible valvular heart disease
- Effects of 5HT — variable effect on vascular tone, depends on the initial tone, BP ↑ if tone low, BP ↓ if tone high
  — mild hyperglycaemia
- Effects of bradykinin — vasodilation and hypotension
  — increased capillary permeability
  — bronchoconstriction

Assessment
- Clinical history and examination
- Serum proteins—exchange of tumour for liver may be reflected in a low protein concentration
- Blood sugar

Preparation
- One hour preoperatively infuse aprotinin (a kallikrein trypsin inhibitor) at a rate of 50 000 units per hour
- Methotrimeprazine (2.5–5.0 mg i.v.) has been suggested to be the anti-5HT drug of choice

Anaesthesia
- Sedative premedication
- Smooth induction/intubation—local anaesthetic to vocal cords and trachea
- Vecuronium or cisatracurium for relaxation
- Fentanyl, alfentanil or phenoperidine is satisfactory
- Octreotide (somatostatin) infusion
- Aprotinin, antihistamines and 5HT antagonists
- Monitor the ECG, intra-arterial pressure, CVP, blood gases and electrolytes intra-operatively.

AVOID
- Morphine—releases 5HT and histamine
- Suxamethonium—fasciculations/raised intra-abdominal pressure may cause the release of hormone from the tumour
- D-tubocurarine—hypotension, histamine release and bronchoconstriction
- Catecholamines

DERMATOLOGICAL PROBLEMS

Actopy
Eczema, asthma, and hayfever: the skin lesions do not present an anaesthetic problem, other than that the siting of intravenous infusions which may be restricted. Atopic patients, however, are thought to be at a greater risk from adverse reactions.

Burns
See p. 165

Epidermolysis bullosa
This is a rare disorder in which blisters form in response to mild trauma to the skin and mucous membranes. Scarring may occur.

Precautions should be taken to avoid trauma—avoid endotracheal intubation if possible. A hydrocortisone-soaked swab should be placed between the face and the mask and only gentle pressure used to maintain a gas tight fit. Porphyria is associated with this condition.

SUMMARY

Index of disease processes with their major 'anaesthesia'-orientated functional defects.

Acromegaly:	Difficult intubation complications
	Glucose intolerance
Acute intermittent porphyria:	Adverse reaction to certain drugs
Addison's disease:	Low cardiac output
	Inability to respond to stress
	Low glucose level
Allergy:	Adverse reaction to some drugs
Anaemia:	Reduced oxygen carriage
Ankylosing spondylitis:	Difficult intubation
Anxiety/depression/psychosis:	Possible drug interactions
	Possible reduced ability to cooperate
Aortic incompetence:	Fixed cardiac output
Aortic stenosis:	Fixed cardiac output
Atrial fibrillation/flutter:	Associated with ischaemic heart disease, thyrotoxicosis, rheumatic heart disease
	Low cardiac output
	— Inadequate contractility
	— Inefficient heart rate
Bronchiectasis:	Lower airway disease
	— Excess secretions
Bronchitis:	Lower airway disease
	— Excess secretions
Bronchopleural fistula:	Lower airway disease

	— Leak
	— Excess secretions
Bullous disorders:	Skin and mucous membranes at risk
Burns:	Possible low cardiac output
	— Inadequate preload (low blood volume)
	— Inadequate contractility (electrolyte imbalance)
	Reduced oxygen carriage
	Increased risk of renal failure
	Altered metabolic state
	Possible upper-airway access dificulty/trauma
Carcinoid syndrome:	Abnormal vasomotor control
	— Variable vascular tone
Christmas disease:	Disorder of coagulation
Congenital heart disease:	Cyanosis
	— Failure of oxygenation (right → left shunt)
	Low cardiac output
	— inefficient circulation path within the heart
	Acyanosis
	— Excess pulmonary flow may lead to pulmonary hypertension
	Low cardiac output
	Inadequate contractility
Conn's syndrome:	Disorder of electrolyte homeostasis
	Possible high cardiac output— increased preload
Cushing's disease:	Possible high cardiac output— increased preload
	Glucose intolerance
	Disorder of electrolyte homoeostasis
Deep vein thrombosis:	Increased risk of thrombosis
Diabetes insipidus:	Low cardiac output—inadequate preload
	Disorder of water homeostasis
Diabetes mellitus:	Glucose intolerance
	Disorder of electrolyte homeostasis
Diffuse intravascular coagulation:	Disorder of coagulation
Drug addiction/intoxication:	Decreased metabolism of drugs
	Australia antigen—hepatitis B
Dystrophia myotonia:	Adverse reaction to some drugs

Emphysema: Lower airway problem—failure of
                                  oxygenation
                                  $\dot{V}/\dot{Q}$ abnormalities
Epilepsy: Adverse reaction to certain drugs
Familial periodic paralysis: Disorder of electrolyte
                                  homeostasis
                                  Abnormally responsive receptors
                                  (neuromuscular junction)
Haemophilia: Disorder of coagulation
Heart block: Low cardiac output—inefficient
                                  heart rate
Hyperparathyroidism: Disorder of electrolyte
                                  homoeostasis
                                  — Adverse reaction to some
                                  drugs
                                  If longstanding, skeletal
                                  abnormalities
                                  — Restriction in thoracic cage—
                                  critical ventilatory ability
                                  Renal failure
Hyperpituitarism: See acromegaly, Cushing's
                                  syndrome
Hypertension: Abnormal vasomotor control—
                                  chronically increased tone
Hyperthyroidism: High cardiac output
                                  — Excess adrenergic activity
                                  — Dysrhythmias
Hypoparathyroidism: Disorder of electrolyte
                                  homoeostasis
                                  Upper airway problem—laryngeal
                                  spasm, tetany
Hypopituitarism: Low cardiac output—inadequate
                                  preload
                                  Disorder of electrolyte
                                  homeostasis
                                  Glucose intolerance—
                                  hypoglycaemia
                                  Inability to respond to stress
Hypothyroidism: Low cardiac output
                                  — Inefficient heart rate
                                  — Reduced contractility
                                  Reduced ability to metabolise
                                  drugs
                                  Reduced ability to respond to
                                  stress
Hypothermia: Low cardiac output
                                  — Inefficient heart rate
                                  — Reduced contractility
                                  — Dysrhythmias

	Reduced ability to metabolise drugs
	Reduced ability to respond to stress
Intestinal obstruction:	Low cardiac output
	— Inadequate preload
	Disorder of electrolyte homeostasis
Ischaemic heart disease:	Low cardiac output
	— Inadequate contractility
	— Inefficient heart rate (dysrhythmias)
Jaundice:	Increased risk of renal failure
Meningitis:	Increased sensitivity to some drugs
	— Deranged blood/brain barrier
Mental retardation:	Possible lack of cooperation
Mitral incompetence:	Fixed cardiac output
	Dysrhythmias
Mitral stenosis:	Fixed cardiac output
	Dysrhythmias
Mutliple sclerosis:	Adverse reaction to some drugs
	Deranged blood/brain barrier
Muscular dystrophy:	Increased sensivity to some drugs (thiopentone, suxamethonium)
Myasthenia gravis:	Abnormally responsive receptors
	Critical ventilatory ability
	Lower airway problem
	— Excess drug-induced secretions
Myasthenic syndrome:	Increased sensivity to some drugs
	Abnormally responsive receptors
Osteomalacia:	Skeletal problem
Paget's disease:	Skeletal problem
	Abnormal vasomotor control
	— Chronically decreased peripheral resistance
	Heart failure (rare)
Parkinsonism:	Possible drug interactions
	Critical ventilatory ability
Pericarditis (constrictive):	Fixed cardiac output/Fixed stroke volume
Peripheral arterial disease:	Abnormal vasomotor control/Fixed tone
	(Associated with ischaemic heart disease)
Peripheral neuropathology:	Increased sensitivity to certain drugs
	— Abnormally responsive receptors

	Possible critical ventilatory ability
	Possible abnormal vasomotor control/Variable tone
Phaeochromocytoma:	Abnormal vasomotor control
	— Variable tone (excess adrenergic activity)
Pneumonia:	High cardiac output
	— Tachycardia (pyrexia)
	Lower airway problem
	— Excess secretions
	Failure of oxygenation/$\dot{V}/\dot{Q}$ abnormality
Pneumothorax/cyst/bulla:	Possible critical ventilatory ability
Poliomyelitis:	Possible critical ventilatory ability
	Possible electrolyte disturbance in the acute stages in association with the use of suxamethonium (hyperkalaemia)
Pulmonary embolism:	Low cardiac output
	— Inadequate preload to left heart
	Failure of oxygenation
	$\dot{V}/\dot{Q}$ abnormality
Renal failure:	Variable cardiac output
	— Increased or decreased preload
	Disorder of electrolyte homeostasis
Rheumatoid arthritis:	Skeletal problems
	Reduced ventilatory ability
	Possible inadequate response to stress (secondary to drug therapy)
Scleroderma:	Upper airway problem (intubation difficulty)
	Possible critical ventilatory ability
Sickle cell disease:	Oxygen carriage disorder
	Abnormally at risk from haemolysis
Thalassaemia:	Abnormally at risk from haemolysis
Von Willebrand's disease:	Disorder of haemostasis

3. Considerations for procedures requiring anaesthesia

EMERGENCY SURGERY

Dangers
- Incomplete history including drug therapy or allergies
- Incomplete biochemical, cardiological and radiological examination
- Patient's condition is progressive, not static
- Gastric stasis—danger of regurgitation

Special action to take
Obtain as full a history and examination as possible in the circumstances. Look for 'medic-alert' bracelets and warning cards. Anticipate exaggerated responses to drugs, e.g. hypotension. Balance the risk of anaesthesia and surgery against the need for immediate surgery (e.g. stomach probably empty if trauma occurred 4 h after a meal; however, stomach may still be full 24 h later if trauma occured immediately after food). Is the surgery so urgent? Urgent need for surgery may deny the opportunity to delay surgery and allow time for spontaneous gastric emptying. The stomach may be emptied by the use of a stomach tube (not 100% reliable). Use a rapid-sequence induction technique, i.e. preoxygenation, induction agent, cricoid pressure, rapid intubation following suxamethonium (or rocuronium). Insert at least one large bore i.v. line.

ANAESTHESIA FOR NEUROSURGERY

There are general considerations which are common to most intracranial procedures: these include posture, control of blood pressure and avoidance of air embolism.

EFFECT OF POSTURE

Supine
The supine position is least likely to cause cardio-respiratory problems. The pooling of blood in dependent parts is reduced and there is no compression of the abdomen and hence the inferior vena cava (assuming the absence of gross obestity or an intra-abdominal mass). The alveolar dead space is minimal when horizontal and the risk of gas embolism is low.

Prone
Special attention must be paid to the protection of the eyes and face, and to the positioning of the head and neck. Support must be provided under the chest and pelvis so that the abdomen is not compressed with resulting pressure on the inferior vena cava and splinting of the diaphragm. Positive pressure ventilation using an armoured (reinforced) tracheal tube is mandatory in the prone position for all surgical procedures.

Sitting position
The cardiovascular system must be carefully monitored during the transition from the horizontal to the sitting position (risk of acute hypotension) and this change in position should be performed slowly. Pooling of blood occurs in dependent limbs. Air embolism is more likely in the sitting position. Some neurosurgical units use 'G' suits over the lower half of the body to aid central venous filling.

GAS EMBOLISM

This is caused by gas bubbles entering the circulation when a vessel with an intraluminal pressure lower than atmospheric pressure is held open. This occurs most commonly to vessels in bony channels and therefore to the venous sinuses within the skull. A small volume of gas may go unnoticed, although Doppler sensors over the praecordium can detect very small amounts (0.25 ml). Larger volumes cause disturbances in respiratory rhythm and may lead to a complete failure of cardiac output due to the heart's inability to pump froth. If air reaches the left side of the heart. (e.g. via an unrecognised small atrial septal defect), even a small bubble may cause irreversible damage, e.g. cerebral or myocardial infarction. The sitting position should be avoided whenever possible. Flooding the operation site with saline will prevent the ingress of air, but may make surgery more difficult. Bone wax may be used to seal bone surfaces. Praecordial monitoring is mandatory in the sitting position. A 'mill-wheel' murmur may be heard through a stethoscope if gas is present in the heart (this is really too late); a Doppler sensor will identify the embolus much earlier. A sudden fall in end tidal CO_2 is a useful early sign.

In case of surgical gas embolism, the surgical site should be flooded with saline, venous pressure should be increased (tipping the table head down is usually impossible, and very unpopular with the surgeon) by using PEEP or a 'G' suit. The inspired gas should be 100% O_2 (N_2O will enlarge the size of air bubbles) and external cardiac compression may be necessary. It is said that gas can be aspirated from the heart via a central venous line. This manoeuvre may be facilitated by turning the patient into the left lateral position (which may be difficult) so that the right side of the heart is uppermost. This reduces the likelihood of the gas bubble passing into the pulmonary circulation. If major embolus occurs early in the procedure the operation should be abandoned.

THE PATIENT WITH RAISED INTRACRANIAL PRESSURE (ICP)

Causes include increased CSF volume (e.g. hydrocephalus); increased brain volume (e.g. tumour, oedema, head injury); increased intracranial blood volume (e.g. venous congestion, arterial dilatation); hypoxaemia and hypercarbia (e.g. respiratory obstruction, respiratory depression); subarachnoid and extradural haemorrhage.

Any increase in one component within the skull must be followed by a reduction in another for the pressure to remain constant. Initially, volume changes displace CSF until a critical point is reached beyond which small changes in volume produce large changes in pressure. Symptoms and signs of raised ICP include nausea, vomiting, headaches, drowsiness, bradycardia, hypotension and papilloedema. ICP is increased by hypercarbia, suxamethonium, halothane and enflurane, but not by isoflurane or desflurane. Propofol, thiopentone, hyperventilation and dehydration reduce ICP. Opioids may increase ICP secondary to respiratory depression unless ventilation is supported.

Maintenance of cerebral perfusion
Cerebral perfusion pressure (mean arterial pressure – intracranial pressure) is the most important cardiovascular factor in patients with raised ICP.
The following should be avoided:
• Venous congestion
• Coughing, straining or vomiting
• Overhydration
• Raised intrathoracic pressure
• Systemic arterial hypotension
• Cerebral arterial vasodilatation due to anaesthetic agents
• Increased P_aCO_2
• Hypoxia

Preparation for anaesthesia
Dehydrate brain tissue by limiting fluid intake and by specific hyperosmolar agents. The use of mannitol should be restricted to the period immediately prior to surgery to avoid a rebound phenomenon leading to a rise in intracranial pressure associated with the movement of agent into the brain tissue. Steroids reduce intracranial pressure by reducing oedema associated with tumours, trauma and hypoxia. Prior to surgery a ventricular drain may be inserted to reduce the dangers associated with severely raised intracranial pressures. Induced hypotension and cooling have been used to facilitate difficult surgery.

Essential points of management
- Dehydrating agents
- Controlled ventilation
- Avoiding venous congestion
- Avoiding excessive use of volatile anaesthetic agents

Postoperative care
- Ensure that relaxation is reversed and adequate spontaneous ventilation is established prior to extubation
- Monitor CSF pressure
- If ventilation is controlled, monitor end tidal carbon dioxide concentration
- Monitor neurological function

THE PATIENT WITH NORMAL INTRACRANIAL PRESSURE

Reasons for intracranial surgery include cerebral artery aneurysm, vascular anomaly and other non-obstructive lesions. Problems associated with patients with cerebral aneurysms include possible hypertension and instability of blood pressure. A brain which is too flaccid (due to dehydration) may remove support from the aneurysm and cause further bleeding.

Essential points of management
- Avoid any rise in $P_a CO_2$
- Avoid a rise in venous pressure
- Avoid hypoxia
- Avoid ventilatory obstruction (care with PEEP)
- Avoid hypertension
- Minimise the use of inhalational agents

A short period of intense hypotension may be required during the clipping of an aneurysm; this can be achieved using, for example, sodium nitroprusside.

OPHTHALMIC SURGERY

SPECIAL FACTORS

1. Control of intra-ocular pressure (IOP) (normal 25 mmHg). Many of the factors affecting intracranial pressure also effect intra-ocular pressure. IOP is increased by suxamethonium, ketamine, atropine (not i.v.), coughing, straining, vomiting and hypertension.
2. Certain drugs used in anaesthesia may affect pupil size. Miotics, e.g. anticholinesterases, carbachol and pilocarpine, cause constriction of the pupil. In acute glaucoma a reduction in IOP results as the angle of the anterior chamber is cleared of the pupillary muscle. Mydriatics (e.g. atropine, hyoscine, cyclopentylate) can precipitate acute glaucoma in those patients at risk. Intravenous atropine in normal dosage is not a hazard in this respect.

3. Aschner's oculo-cardiac reflex (afferent fibres in ophthalmic branch of the trigeminal nerve, efferent fibres in the vagus). Bradycardia and cardiac arrest are associated with traction on the eyeball. The incidence may be reduced by atropine and by drugs with atropine-like effects, particularly if combined with relaxation.

EMERGENCY OPEN-EYE SURGERY IN THE PRESENCE OF FULL STOMACH

Intubation of the trachea and controlled ventilation are normal practice. Suxamethonium used to facilitate intubation during induction of general anaesthesia may lead to vitreous prolapse. The risk of vomiting, with the risk of inhaling gastric contents, must be reduced as this may also be associated with loss of vitreous. One the other hand, the risk of loss of sight in one eye must be equated with the potential risk to life from pulmonary aspiration of gastric contents. Rocuronium is used instead of suxamethonium in some centres for these patients.

EAR, NOSE AND THROAT

AURAL SURGERY

Minor procedures on the external ear or the insertion of grommets in a child do not necessitate any special precautions. A technique that involves spontaneously breathing with a facemask or laryngeal mask is appropriate in most cases.

Special factors in major middle-ear surgery
1. Control of bleeding. This includes use of a vasoconstrictor by the surgeon, avoidance of venous congestion by the anaesthetist and control of blood pressure.
2. N_2O diffusion into air spaces. A rise in pressure occurs as N_2O diffuses into the middle ear. If a tympanic membrane graft has been inserted it may become dislodged. The administration of nitrous oxide should cease at least 30 min before the graft is applied. If 100% oxygen is administered following the use of nitrous oxide it is possible to produce a negative pressure within the middle ear cavity. Ventilation with an oxygen/air mixture is recommended to prevent pressure gradients developing.
3. Intra-operative communication with the patient is usually reserved for those who are undergoing surgery of the ossicles or labyrinthine ablation and is now rare. It is more common to use evoked responses. Auditory stimulation results in a change in the electrical discharge on the surface of the cerebral cortex (an evoked response), and can be used to test auditory function during anaesthesia.
4. Avoidance of neuromuscular blocking agents allows facial movements to be seen, should the drill irritate the facial nerve.

NASAL SURGERY

These operations are usually short and straightforward, e.g. polypectomy. Patients with a fractured nose may have suffered a recent head injury. The nose is very vascular and the application of a topical vasoconstrictor is valuable. The popularity of topical cocaine has waned and commercially available drops or spray (e.g. oxymetazoline) are more commonly used. Direct injection of 1 in 200 000 adrenaline is favoured by some surgeons.

If there has been bleeding from the nose, beware the risk of swallowed blood. Use a rapid sequence induction technique. Intubation of the trachea is required to protect the airway from blood. A pharnygeal pack is valuable, but remember to remove it at the end. Extubate in the lateral position and avoid pressure on the nose from face masks.

Access to the pituitary gland is gained through the nose (transnasal approach). This may be a lengthy procedure. Hormone replacement may be required at the end of the procedure, e.g. pitressin, hydrocortisone, thyroxine.

PHARYNGEAL/LARYNGEAL SURGERY

Preservation of the airway and sharing it with the surgeon are principal considerations.

Tonsillectomy
Tracheal intubation is performed following induction of anaesthesia and a muscle relaxant. An oral RAE tracheal tube is useful as it is easily positioned centrally between the jaws of the mouth gag. A nasal tube may be used in adults (not children). The patient may breathe spontaneously or be ventilated. The head is positioned in extension with a roll or pad beneath the shoulders if extension is inadequate. Bradycardia may occur during dissection, particularly of the adenoids. Blood loss can be deceptive. Extubation should be performed with the patient in the lateral, head-down position. This procedure may be performed as a day case with careful patient selection.

Post-tonsillectomy bleeding
There may be evidence of significant loss of blood (e.g. hypotension, tachycardia, sweating, peripheral cyanosis). Blood loss may be much greater than external appearance because large quantities of blood may have been swallowed.

Essential management principles include:
1. Establish an intravenous infusion and obtain blood for transfusion. Fully resuscitate prior to induction.
2. Use the lateral head-down position; clear pharynx of blood clots.

3. Administer 100% oxygen.
4. Induce anaesthesia. Either an inhalational induction using halothane or sevoflurane in oxygen or an intravenous induction with a reduced dose of intravenous agent (etomidate is suitable), suxamethonium, and cricoid pressure.
5. Intubate with a cuffed tube.
6. At the end of the operation, some authors suggest removing blood from the stomach by passing a large-bore nasogastric tube and washing out the stomach.

Laryngoscopic examination or microsurgery
Inhalational anaesthesia with halothane or sevoflurane and spontaneous ventilation using 100% oxygen may be required. Alternatively, intravenous induction, muscle relaxant and controlled ventilation through a narrow (e.g. 6 mm) cuffed tube or alternatively a Pollard, Carden or Coplans tube is used.
Intravenous induction, muscle relaxant and controlled ventilation using a venturi or high-frequency jet ventilator is used in some centres. Anaesthesia is maintained using TIVA.

DENTAL SURGERY

ANAESTHESIA FOR OUTPATIENT DENTAL SURGERY

Contraindications
1. Significant cardiovascular disease
2. Significant respiratory disease (upper or lower respiratory tract)
3. Certain drugs, e.g. anticoagulants
4. Endocrine disease which is not stable on treatment, e.g. brittle diabetes mellitus, pituitary disease
5. Miscellaneous: porphyria, 1st trimester of pregnancy, abnormal haemoglobinopathies including thalassaemia and sickle cell disease.

Indications
1. Infection
2. Failed local anaesthesia
3. Age—young children
4. Allergy to local anaesthetic agents
5. Mental retardation
6. Neurological disease associated with involuntary movement
7. Multiple extractions in different quadrants of the mouth

Additional considerations
• Competent adult escort home essential
• Unprepared or incompletely investigated patients are unsuitable
• Patients with an unstable medical condition are unsuitable as day cases

- Postoperative swelling in the mouth and airway
- Appropriate supply of analgesia

Sedation and local anaesthesia
Local anaesthesia alone is used for many outpatient procedures. The addition of sedation is useful to reduce discomfort for patients with dental phobia. Intravenous diazepam or midazolam combined with the injection of a local anaesthetic agent is a common technique.

Patients should be supine during treatment. The glottic reflex may be obtunded and reduced muscle tone may lead to respiratory obstruction. The aim should be to maintain verbal contact with the patient throughout. Airway safety is then assured. Patients can generally leave the surgery 90 min after injection. All patients who have received sedation must be accompanied by a responsible adult and must not control machinery or drive a car for at least 24 h.

Relative analgesia is a technique whereby a 20–30% mixture of nitrous oxide in oxygen is administered via a nasal mask. Verbal contact is maintained. The injection of local anaesthetic in the anxious individual is facilitated.

General anaesthesia technique
In children an inhalational induction using oxygen, nitrous oxide and halothane or sevoflurane is usually routine. In adults intravenous induction using propofol or methohexitone is common. The position for surgery has received much consideration. The supine position is safest because the danger associated with a severe fall in blood pressure in a more upright position, is less. It is more difficult to control the patency of the airway, however. The airway requires protection from dental debris and irrigation fluids and this can be secured by tracheal intubation and placement of an oral pack.

Recovery may appear to be rapid. However, approximately 10% of patients feel sleepy the next day. EEG changes may still be detected even though performance at tests of skill has returned to pre-anaesthetic levels. The patient requires to be escorted home, and should not operate or control machinery, drive a car, or take sedatives, tranquillisers, hypnotics or alcohol for at least 24 h. Tests of recovery are generally of little value and certainly do not offer more information than the unsophisticated test of ability to walk unaided.

Inpatient dental anaesthetics are given to patients whose medical condition makes them unsuitable for outpatient treatment, e.g. pregnancy, cardiac disease, respiratory disease. Nasal intubation is commonly performed in order to facilitate surgical access. Damage to the nasal mucosa with severe haemorrhage may occur or infected debris may be pushed down the nasal passages into the larynx. The diameter of a nasal tube is less than an equivalent oral tube in the same patient; this increases the resistance to flow.

Other factors of particular interest include the danger of bleeding in the upper airway and cardiac dysrhythmias due to dental manipulation. The risk of dysrhythmias is increased by spontaneous ventilation (raised $P_a CO_2$), and the use of halothane.

ANAESTHESIA FOR MAXILLO-FACIAL SURGERY

Intubation may be required in the presence of possible bleeding and oedema. There is a risk of meningitis in those patients with a fractured base of skull. The mandible, maxilla, zygoma and floor of the mouth may be involved in the surgery; therefore intubation is required. Intubation should be performed with the patient breathing spontaneously if it is likely to be difficult. Alternatively, an awake fibreoptic intubation technique under local analgesia has much to recommend it. Anatomical deformity resulting from tumour, trauma or certain well-defined syndromes such as Treacher–Collins are all possible. The choice between nasal and oral intubation depends on the site of the surgery and possible invasion of the airway by tumour or oedema, or gross deformity due to trauma. Recovery presents special problems. If the jaws have been wired together, airway control may be difficult and vomiting becomes particularly hazardous. The use of an antiemetic is advisable. It is advisable to leave a nasopharyngeal airway in situ during recovery and to have wire cutters available in case severe airway obstruction occurs.

Fully assess airway and intubation potential carefully preoperatively. The patency of the airway must be protected— reinforced (armoured) endotracheal tube, airway and a mouth prop or dental ring well secured. The eyes must be protected. Intravenous infusions should be sited so that they are easily accessible and away from the operating site. Coaxial circuits are useful because they reduce the bulk of tubing, although modern lightweight tubing is often used. Integrity of anaesthetic circuit should be easily confirmed even when hidden under drapes, e.g. monitoring of expired gas or measurement of airway pressure or preferably both.

ANAESTHESIA FOR SURGERY OF THE HEAD AND NECK

Parotid surgery

Spontaneous ventilation permits the use of a nerve stimulator to confirm identification of the facial nerve. An alternative technique is to use a controlled ventilation and a muscle relaxant with a rapid recovery profile (e.g. mivacurium), the effect of which can be allowed to wane at the appropriate time. Control of blood pressure may be required. Venous oozing can be controlled by a 10° head-up tilt.

Plastic surgery
Control of blood pressure may be required. For surgery involving superficial structures a basal sedation/local anaesthetic technique may be used (e.g. a benzodiazepine). The patency and safety of the airway is always of prime importance and the maintenance of verbal contact is essential.

ANAESTHESIA FOR SURGERY OF THE NECK

POSTERIOR APPROACH

Decompression of cervical cord, stabilisation of diseased or traumatised vertebrae and repair of meningomyelocoele are all performed via this route. There may be immobility of cervical spine with difficult intubation. An orthopaedic fixation frame enveloping chest and head will also result in a difficult intubation. There is a danger of cord compression with neck flexion (in rheumatoid patients) and neck extension (certain cervical fractures).

Management
If a difficult intubation is anticipated:
• Anxiolytic-type premedication—Consider awake intubation
• A full set of aids to intubation should be available, as should equipment for cricothyroid puncture
• Armoured (reinforced) endotracheal tubes—to avoid kinking
• IPPV
• Prone position—avoid compression of abdomen, neck, eyes and nose

ANTERIOR APPROACH TO THE NECK

Thyroid surgery
The patient should be euthyroid. Identify patients at risk by clinical signs, e.g. tachycardia, atrial fibrillation or heart failure, and biochemical tests. Tracheal compression may cause intubation difficulties. Tracheomalacia may lead to postoperative tracheal collapse. Tracheal compression may also result from postoperative haemorrhage. Recurrent laryngeal nerve damage may lead to hoarseness or stridor and re-intubation may be necessary. Check vocal cord movement at time of extubation.

Excision of parathyroids
Measure plasma calcium preoperatively and also intra-operatively. In the postoperative period a calcium infusion may be required to

maintain blood calcium level and avoid muscle spasms. Check plasma calcium frequently postoperatively to prevent increased cardiac irritability leading to ventricular fibrillation.

Tracheostomy

As an acute emergency procedure see p. 121.

If the upper airway is a problem then the routine described on p. 82 should be followed to ensure safety during the intubation sequence. The entire procedure may be carried out using a regional block or by local infiltration.

Assuming tracheal intubation is possible, surgical exposure of the trachea, and construction of the tracheostome, is followed by careful withdrawal of the endotracheal tube to a point just above the opening. A sterile tracheostomy tube is then connected to a sterile set of respiratory hose compatible with the breathing system in use. Do not draw the tracheal tube out through the vocal cords until the airway is guaranteed via the tracheostomy tube in case there is a problem. The tracheal tube can then be advanced again to re-establish ventilation.

Percutaneous dilational tracheostomy has become a routine procedure in the intensive care unit. Here, an incision is made in the neck below the cricoid ring. The tissues are parted by blunt dissection and any vessels tied. A needle is then inserted into the trachea, and a guide wire is passed through the needle. The needle is removed and dilators of increasing size are passed until the tracheostomy tube can be inserted.

Laryngectomy

Tumour may encroach on the airway, making intubation hazardous or even impossible. Great care should be taken with the induction of anaesthesia should the patency of the larynx be in doubt. A preliminary tracheostomy may be necessary; surgically this is less than satisfactory. Direct access to the airways is lost when the surgeons excise the larynx. A separate set of sterile respiratory hose should be available.

Cervical spine surgery

Similar problems may be encountered to those described for the posterior approach to the cervical spine. Distraction of the cervical spine is usually necessary to enable the insertion of a bone graft to span adjacent vertebrae. The skull calipers provide a traction point.

SURGERY TO THE CHEST

ANAESTHESIA FOR SURGERY INVOLVING THE RIB CAGE

- Correction of pectus excavatum/carinatum
- Fixation of flail chest

- Derangement of rib cage associated with kyphoscoliosis (see next section)

In each condition the integrity of the chest wall is abnormal. Surgery may result in an increase in vital capacity and an improvement in cardiac performance. Fixation of a flail segment should improve respiratory function.

Management
1. Endotracheal intubation and controlled ventilation to ensure adequate pulmonary ventilation
2. Postoperative analgesia is selected to avoid ventilatory depression

ANAESTHESIA FOR SURGERY OF THE THORACIC SPINE

Severe spinal curvature reduces both the vital capacity and total lung volume (restrictive disease). The lung volumes are further decreased with increasing spinal curvature (reduced FRC), leading to a reduction in the ventilation-to-perfusion ratio with arterial hypoxaemia and hypercarbia.

Preoperative identification and full investigation of pulmonary and cardiac disease and institution of correct control therapy are essential. Patients may be chronically hypoxaemic and intubation may be difficult. Patients must therefore be preoxygenated and controlled ventilation during anaesthesia will be necessary. Controlled ventilation may also be required in the postoperative period.

Surgery for kyphoscoliosis (Harrington operation)
The intention is to reduce and to arrest progress of the spinal curvature by vertebral fusion and internal fixation using metal rods. The operation is extensive and there may be considerable blood loss during surgery and in the postoperative period. Blood loss may be reduced by using an appropriate posture and by keeping the mean intrathoracic pressure low. On the other hand, although induced arterial hypotension may be helpful, it may exacerbate the bleeding if this is primarily due to venous oozing (congested epidural veins).

The prone position may lead to a rise in intra-abdominal pressure, thereby reducing or preventing venous return from the lower limbs, with increased blood loss. Communication with the patient during anaesthesia may be considered desirable to detect cord damage during traction on the vertebrae, although evoked potentials are more often used in current practice.

ANAESTHESIA FOR PULMONARY SURGERY

Pulmonary resection occasionally may lead to right ventricular failure associated with a sudden rise in pulmonary vascular resistance and also to a reduction in pulmonary performance leading to repiratory failure.

General considerations
- Careful preoperative assessment of cardiorespiratory reserve
- Maintenance of gaseous exchange during surgery on the lungs or main airways
- Control of secretions
- Postoperative respiratory complications

Resection of lung tissue

Preoperative assessment
- Medical history, including character and amount of sputum and an assessment of dyspnoea
- General clinical examination
- Pulmonary function tests
- Blood gas analysis
- Exercise tolerance
- Clinical assessment of right ventricular function and pulmonary hypertension, including right ventricular strain (ECG)

Theoretically the likely effect of resection of diseased lung on pulmonary artery pressures may be determined during cardiac catheterisation by occluding the arterial supply to the diseased lung.

Management
- Endobronchial intubation and one-lung anaesthesia
- Lateral or Parry Brown position
- Assessment of the adequacy of one lung, if there is doubt, by clamping the pulmonary artery to the diseased lung. Reduction of the shunt fraction should lead to a rise in P_aO_2.
- After pulmonary surgery a chest drain, sometimes two, is attached to an underwater seal in order to facilitate pulmonary expansion and pleural cavity drainage. Following pneumonectomy care must be taken not to reduce the pressure in the pleural cavity lest cardiac function is compromised by displacement of the mediastinum. If a chest drain is inserted it is clamped off and only released, once an hour, to determine the amount of postoperative bleeding.
- Where possible a policy of extubation with spontaneous ventilation should be followed. This prevents the application of high airway pressure or the tip of the endotracheal tube reopening the sutured, or stapled, bronchial stump.

TRACHEAL RESECTION

Tracheal resection is carried out for a stricture or tumour. An inhalational induction should be used to preserve spontaneous ventilation. An armoured tube is advisable. Passage of the tube using a fibreoptic bronchoscope under direct vision may be required. A stricture or tumour may permit only a small-diameter endotracheal tube to be passed. If intubation with an endotracheal tube fails it may be possible to pass a bronchoscope past the narrowing and ventilate using a venturi. A muscle relaxant may be used after the airway has been secured. During surgery the distal portion of the trachea is intubated once the resection has been performed. The posterior aspect of the trachea is sutured so that the distal segment is intubated via the proximal segment. The suturing of the anastomosis is then completed. Cardiopulmonary bypass has been used to facilitate tracheal resection.

Spontaneous ventilation should be resumed postoperatively to avoid trauma to the tracheal suture line by the endotracheal tube. Excessive coughing during extubation may damage the tracheal suture line.

DRAINAGE OF AN EMPYEMA

A history of copious purulent sputum suggests a connection between an empyema and the tracheobronchial tree. Precautions must therefore be taken to prevent entry of pus to the airways.

The classic approach is to use local anaesthesia in the sitting position for rib resection and drainage of the abscess cavity. If general anaesthesia is to be used, the requirements are a smooth induction with the empyema in a dependent position. Spontaneous ventilation should be continued until the main airways are intubated and isolated with a double lumen tube or a bronchial blocker. The patient may then be turned so that the empyema is uppermost and IPPV can be instituted. The abscess cavity is normally drained by a large-bore tube. Bronchoscopy, using spontaneous ventilation, is indicated if a bronchopleural fistula is thought to exist and if surgical intervention is considered.

PLEURECTOMY/EXCISION OF BULLAE OR CYSTS

General considerations
- Possible increase in tension in an existing pneumothorax or cyst
- Air leak in the postoperative stage

Management
- If there is no chest drain in situ then facilities for the insertion of a chest drain should be immediately available.

- Endobronchial intubation: IPPV may lead to an increase in tension within the pneumothorax or cyst and therefore spontaneous ventilation is preferred until isolation of the involved lung is assured. Nitrous oxide should be avoided.
- IPPV should be avoided postoperatively to reduce the likelihood of an air leak.

TRANSTHORACIC HIATUS HERNIA REPAIR

Preoxygenation followed by cricoid pressure during intubation is essential to prevent regurgitation of gastric contents. Endobronchial intubation is not essential but one-lung anaesthesia improves surgical access. A left-sided double-lumen tube, which is easier to position, is frequently used. A nasogastric tube is normally inserted because it aids the surgeon during mobilisation of the oesophagus, but may be withdrawn at the end of the operation.

OESOPHAGEAL RESECTION

The patient may be in a state of chronic undernutrition and so preoperative parenteral nutrition should be considered. Rehydration will be necessary if dysphagia is severe—several litres of colloid and crystalloid may be necessary. Operative management is the same as that described for hiatus hernia repair with the added problem of prolonged surgery.

Tracheo-oesophageal fistula (TOF)

Tracheo-oesophageal fistulae are usually of the congenital variety although fistulae can occur as a result of neoplasia, trauma, or prolonged endotracheal intubation. The congenital variety may be associated with cardiac defects (Fig. 3.1).

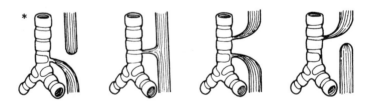

* Most common

Fig 3.1   Four configurations of tracheo-oesophageal fistula

Management of the neonate with congenital TOF

Preparation
Any chest infection associated with contamination of the airway with feed and/or saliva must be treated before surgery. A nasogastric tube of the double-lumen Replogle type should be passed to allow cleansing and emptying of the oesophageal pouch. Hydration should be maintained intravenously. X-ray investigation is required to determine the position of the fistula. (TOF in the neonate is not considered an emergency procedure and the preparation as described above should be carried out.)

Anaesthesia
The neonate should be intubated, with a single-lumen tube, whilst breathing spontaneously. Ventilatory movements will indicate whether the fistula has been intubated, in which case the tube must be repositioned. Spontaneous respiration may be maintained until the chest is opened or, alternatively, a tentative manual inflation of the lungs may be performed to assess the ability to inflate the lungs and observe whether stomach inflation occurs. All other matters pertaining to neonatal anaesthesia must, of course, be considered.

Tracheo-oesophageal fistula in the adult should be managed in a similar way to that described for the patient with a bronchopleural leak in that a double-lumen tube should be used to isolate the lung with the leak. Surgical access is improved and contamination of the lungs with oesophageal contents is limited.

ANAESTHESIA FOR SURGERY OF THE GREAT VESSELS (NOT INVOLVING CARDIOPULMONARY BYPASS)

Coarctation of the aorta
Bleeding from the chest wall can be severe (notched ribs, due to tortuous blood vessels, reflect the development of an extensive collateral circulation). Cross-clamping of the aorta may lead to a rise in blood pressure followed by a marked fall when the clamps are removed. Though severe hypotension may occur immediately after the clamps are removed, postoperative hypertension is also possible and should be treated by sedation, posture and a specific antihypertensive agent if required.

Management
- Monitor blood pressure above and below the coarctation (arm and leg)
- Monitor CVP
- Induction should be designed to maintain the blood pressure
- Prepare for massive blood transfusion
- A hypotensive technique may be considered to reduce bleeding
- Endobronchial intubation with one-lung anaesthesia

Patent ductus arteriosus

During intra-uterine life approximately 80% of the fetal blood ejected into the pulmonary artery is short-circuited into the aorta. During the first 3 weeks of neonatal life the ductus closes permanently. If, however, the patency of the ductus persists then it is usually surgically closed before irreversible pulmonary hypertension occurs.

Pulmonary artery banding

This is a palliative measure designed to reduce the pulmonary artery blood flow and is used in the management of pulmonary hypertension and in the presence of cardiac septal defects with a left-to-right shunt.

Blalock procedure

This is a palliative measure designed to increase pulmonary artery blood flow in order to increase oxygenation in severe pulmonary stenosis and cyanotic congenital heart disease. Systemic blood is allowed to pass, some for a second time, through the pulmonary circulation by the creation of an artificial fistula between the pulmonary and systemic circulations.

For these last three procedures the cardiac output and pressures within the separate cardiac compartments and great vessels should be maintained constant to avoid a disruption in the flow pattern with an increase in hypoxia and myocardial strain.

Ketamine increases pulmonary artery pressure and may alter the amount and even the direction of the flow through the shunt. It may therefore be considered unsuitable in these conditions. In children one-lung anaesthesia is technically difficult and is not therefore usually employed.

ANAESTHESIA FOR SURGERY INVOLVING CARDIOPULMONARY BYPASS (CPB)

- Coronary artery surgery
- Valve replacement
- Repair of anatomical defects

Early techniques (Drew) involved the use of hypothermia to temperatures of 10–15°C. During the cooling process two blood pumps are used: one pumps blood from the left atrium through a heat exchanger into the systemic circulaton and a second pumps blood from the right atrium into the pulmonary artery for oxygenation in the lungs. The method suffers from the prolonged preparatory period with the use of two pumps and multiple cannulation.

1. Partial CPB

Femoral vein	$\rightarrow$	Femoral artery
Left atrium	$\rightarrow$	Aorta
Inferior vena cava	$\rightarrow$	Pulmonary artery

The technique of partial CPB has been used to enable cooling of the whole body. The partial CPB augments the depressed cardiac output and therefore increases the arterial flow.

The technique has also been used to improve oxygenation for patients with severe potentially reversible pulmonary disease (ARDS) although the results are not very encouraging.

2. Full CPB

Superior vena cava	$\rightarrow$		$\rightarrow$ Aorta	
		Oxygenator		
Inferior vena cava	$\rightarrow$		$\rightarrow$ Coronary arteries	

This technique is used routinely for most open-heart surgery—coronary artery cannulation is used during surgery of the aortic valve.

3. Haemodilution

A priming volume is required for the oxygenator and pump and this must be sufficient to provide a reserve of blood (25% of the minute volume flow) which, in the event of a temporary cessation of venous return to the pump, will be available for the patient, thereby reducing the danger of air being drawn into the circuit and causing air embolus. The use of whole blood may be associated with coagulation defects and impaired postoperative lung function. Crystalloid solutions including Hartmann's solution or 5% dextrose are used in modern haemodilution techniques. Gelatin solution may be added. Dilution is limited only by the concomitant reduction in oxygen-carrying capacity. A reduction in blood viscosity, including that associated with hypothermia, can improve venous return and tissue perfusion.

In adults the dilution should not generally reduce packed cell volume below about 30%. Whole blood may be used to prime the oxygenator for use with an infant because the priming volume is much greater than the infant's own blood volume.

4. Control of venous return (to the CPB pump)

This is normally passive by gravity. The operating table is set at a fixed height above the inlet to the pump. Active suction may cause collapse of the veins around the cannulae or the ingress of air.

5. Oxygenators
a. Rotating disc and screen oxygenators effectively disperse blood in oxygen. They are expensive and require a large priming volume.
b. Bubble oxygenators allow oxygen bubbles to pass with the blood through a column, thereby giving rise to a froth. Bubble size is an essential consideration. Large bubbles favour carbon dioxide removal whereas small bubbles are not easily eliminated from the blood. The froth bubbles are largely dissipated on a silicone antifoam surface and remaining bubbles are trapped in the settling reservoirs. Disposable bubble oxygenators which require only a small priming volume are available.
c. Membrane oxygenators use a membrane interface between the blood and oxygen, and mimic the normal relations between blood and gas in the lungs. The duration of bypass can be extended using this method. This may be largely due to the preservation of the plasma proteins which may be destroyed by repeated exposure to a large blood–gas interface.

6. Control of anticoagulation
Heparin (3 mg.kg^{-1}) is given intravenously through a central line. Further doses are administered at intervals according to the activated clotting time (ACT) which is measured at intervals. Most units maintain the ACT at greater than 400 seconds. The blood heparin may be titrated against protamine standards to determine more accurately the required protamine dose. Sometimes the heparin protamine complex is broken down, with resulting prolonged anticoagulation. Loss of fibrinogen may produce a similar effect and should be excluded as a cause of bleeding before giving more protamine.

7. Cardioplegia
Cardiac surgery is easier if the heart is still. Cessation of organised myocardial activity is brought about by perfusing the coronary arteries with a potassium-containing solution. Ischaemic damage to the myocardium can be minimised by bathing the heart in cold saline—care must be taken that local myocardial damage is not caused by ice particles.

8. Hypothermia
Cooling is carried out using the pump so that temperature gradients are minimised.

9. Gas embolism
See p. 83.

10. 'Cardiac' output
A flow from the bypass pump of less than 2.4 $l.m^{-2}.min^{-1}$ tends to cause metabolic acidosis. Tissue perfusion is more dependent upon the peripheral resistance than on the absolute flow rate.

11. Inotropic agents
See p. 153.

12. Mechanical cardiac support
In severe myocardial failure the improvement in coronary perfusion from the use of intra-aortic balloon counterpulsation may result in improved myocardial contractility. The purpose of the intra-aortic balloon is to maintain the diastolic pressure so that an increase in coronary artery flow occurs. The device, a balloon that can be inflated with helium, is positioned in the upper aorta via a femoral artery. It is triggered by the ECG and inflates during diastole; this reduces the egress of blood from the ascending aorta and hence maintains the diastolic pressure. The balloon deflates during systole.

13. Postoperative monitoring
This should include the following:
• Mean arterial pressure
• Central venous pressure
• Left atrial pressure
• Pulmonary artery occlusion pressure
• Cardiac output
• Urinary output
• Clotting studies
• Urea and electrolytes
• ECG
• Arterial gas tensions
• Core and peripheral temperature

ABDOMINAL/PELVIC SURGERY

HERNIORRHAPHY

Inguinal hernias are relatively common, femoral less so. Incisional hernia implies previous surgery. Congenital hernia may be related to the presence of a myopathy and rarely this may carry an increased risk of malignant hyperpyrexia. A hernia developing later in life may be related to a persistent cough associated with chronic bronchitis.

General anaesthesia, local anaesthesia, epidural, spinal or local infiltration may all be used. There are no conditions which are an absolute indication for a particular approach to anaesthesia but clearly respiratory depression and cardiovascular instability must be avoided in patients who have myocardial or pulmonary disease. Infiltration of local anaesthetic agent in the region of the incision has much to commend it for the poor-risk patient.

Omphalocoele, gastroschisis, and diaphragmatic hernia, in which abdominal organs are prolapsed outside the peritoneal cavity, are associated with ventilatory impairment when the extra-abdominal organs are returned to the repaired abdominal cavity. Omphalocoele may lead to peritonitis unless surgically closed and this surgery is urgent. Limitation of pulmonary expansion may lead to hypoxia and cyanosis. The condition is commonly congenital but may result from trauma. Positive pressure ventilation is required and elective postoperative ventilation should be considered.

ABDOMINAL VASCULAR SURGERY

Aortic surgery

Hazards
- Coexisting ischaemic heart disease
- Renal artery involvement
- Friable tissues
- Maintenance of blood volume (may be impossible in the presence of a massive leak)

Management
- Preoperative assessment of cardiovascular function, see p. 42.
- Induction of anaesthesia without cardiovascular depression. A 'G' suit has been found to be useful in maintaining the central blood volume.
- Central venous, peripheral venous and arterial cannulation are required
- Insert a urinary catheter; urine flow being a good indicator of tissue perfusion
- Anticoagulants are administered as requested
- $NaHCO_3$ (50 mmol) may be given before the removal of the femoral artery clamps; this compensates for the washout of acid metabolites from the ischaemic legs
- Postoperative IPPV may be required

Saddle embolectomy

Hazards
- The patient may be very ill, even moribund.
- Patients usually have an arteriopathy and an obvious source of emboli such as valvular heart disease or a recent myocardial infarct.

Management
- Local anaesthesia unless uncooperative. Blood volume should be maintained and supportive measures taken as required.
- The ECG, CVP and blood loss should be monitored.

Renal artery surgery
Renal artery surgery is usually required to relieve a stenosis.

Hazards
- Acute perioperative hypertension may occur.

Management
- Preoperative assessment and antihypertensive therapy are important, the latter should be continued throughout the period of surgery.

Myocardial depression and hypotension should be avoided. Blood volume expansion is the treatment for hypotension. Pressor drugs should be used with great caution and, if required, select the drug to be effective in the presence of the antihypertensive medication. Ketamine and pancuronium may lead to a marked rise in blood pressure. Monitor the ECG, CVP and blood loss; ensure that the blood volume is maintained.

UPPER ABDOMINAL GENERAL SURGERY

This includes surgery to the stomach, bladder, biliary tree, liver, pancreas and small bowel. For oesophageal surgery, see p. 96.

General considerations
- Postoperative ileus—a nasogastric tube will be required, see p. 115.
- Postoperative pain and respiratory complications, see p. 142.
- Electrolyte disturbances may occur due to prolonged vomiting or diarrhoea. These should be corrected before induction.
- Pyloric obstruction may reduce gastric emptying and promote regurgitation during induction of anaesthesia.
- Traction to the vagal fibres in the upper abdomen may lead to bradycardia.

Portal hypertension may lead to haematemesis, with a resulting acute anaemia; liver failure may coexist. Porto-caval anastomosis operations are generally prolonged and usually involve a transthoracic approach.

Open surgical procedures for portal hypertension are less common now with the development of X-ray guided transvenous procedures. Excision of the spleen is usually carried out because of trauma, or for haematological reasons. If platelets are to be administered they should be administered after the splenic artery has been ligated. Pneumococcal vaccination is recommended if the spleen is removed.

Management
An intravenous induction, relaxant, intubation, controlled ventilation technique is recommended. Intravenous fluids are required to compensate for preoperative fluid deprivation and intra-operative losses, which may be considerable if a large surface area of the intestine is exposed or handled excessively. Fluid is lost into the serosa due to the handling ('the third space') and evaporation with additional heat loss.

Liver transplant surgery

Problems
- Impairment of drug metabolism
- Reduced cardiac output after the inferior vena cava is clamped.
- Sudden rapid loss of blood—massive transfusion, p. 121.
- Acidosis resulting from donor liver releasing cold acid perfusate rich in K^+
- Anaemia
- Impairment of hepatic function leading to bleeding and reduced plasma cholinesterase
- Coagulation deficiencies require immediate management
- Blood sugar levels should be closely monitored—there is a risk of hypoglycaemia
- Hypothermia is a common problem

Management
- All drug doses should be adjusted, p. 61.
- IPPV will be required postoperatively
- Renal failure may occur and a diuretic may therefore be required prophylactically during surgery
- Facilities for massive transfusion are essential
- Intensive monitoring is mandatory

Nephrectomy/pyeloplasty/pyelolithotomies

Problems
- The lateral position leads to ventilation perfusion imbalance. Ventilation is biased to the upper lung during IPPV and blood flow to the dependent lung.
- Venal caval compression may reduce venous return and cardiac output.
- Impaired renal function disorder, see p. 55.

Management
If renal function is impaired choose drugs which do not rely on the kidney for elimination.

Renal transplantation

Hazards
- This is normally carried out as a moderately urgent procedure
- Chronic renal failure, p. 55.
- Uraemia/anaemia/hypertension/electrolyte disturbance
- Hypovolaemia and hypokalaemia are possible if the patient has been recently dialysed; overhydration and hyperkalaemia if not

Management
- Avoid drugs which may produce hypotension
- Avoid drugs which are not metabolised and are excreted by the kidneys
- Blood transfusion should be avoided if possible to avoid inducing antibody formation
- Insert a CVP line
- Avoid the likelihood of damage to the shunt or arterio-venous fistula—haemodialysis may still be required

LOWER ABDOMINAL AND PELVIC SURGERY

Procedures include colectomy, anterior resection of sigmoid colon, abdomino-perineal resection, bladder surgery and gynaecological surgery.

Hazards:
- Postoperative ileus
- Abdominal incision, so pain may affect respiration
- Trendelenberg/Lloyd Davies lithotomy positions—p. 111
- Deep vein thrombosis—p. 119

Management
- Combination of general and local anaesthesia is useful.
- Pressure rises within the bowel following neostigmine. An increased risk of leak has been suggested.
- Pethidine may be preferable to morphine.

Perineal surgery
Perineal surgery is eminently suited to local anaesthetic techniques. Circumcision and haemorrhoidectomy are particularly painful procedures and a combination of a local anaesthetic (e.g. caudal block) and a general anaesthetic has been advocated. Dilatation of the anal sphincter can cause dysrhythmias. The lithotomy position, together with a request for headdown tilt, may embarrass respiration and for a prolonged procedure tracheal intubation and IPPV should be used.

Anaesthesia should never be induced in the lithotomy position if the patient is likely to regurgitate, e.g. the third trimester of pregnancy, hiatus hernia or a recent meal. The patient cannot be turned quickly and the patient's airway is therefore at risk.

LIMB SURGERY

Operations on the limbs can be divided into three categories: orthopaedic, vascular and superficial minor surgery. For any of these procedures a local anaesthetic technique is possible.

VASCULAR SURGERY

Vascular surgery of the limbs does not specifically require muscle relaxation and thus neuromuscular blockade is not essential; however, some microvascular procedures may take many hours and a technique that employs tracheal intubation and IPPV using neuromuscular blockade may be preferred. Microvascular surgery is dependent on good tissue perfusion for success, and a Biers block (p. 136) using guanethidine diluted with a local anaesthetic solution may be of value. There may be a transient hypertension on release of the tourniquet.

The patient who requires the construction of arterio-venous fistula will require the preparation and management that is described for patients with chronic renal failure, p. 55.

The most common vascular surgery of the legs is stripping, tying or avulsing varicosities. It usually requires the patient to be in the Trendelenberg position. Head-down tilt is associated with diaphragmatic splinting and respiratory embarrassment and IPPV should be considered. IPPV is required if the patient is to be prone for ligation of varicosities on the posterior aspect of the legs.

ORTHOPAEDIC SURGERY

Orthopaedic surgery involving the more distal portions of the limbs can be carried out using an airway and mask or laryngeal mask. Surgery on the shoulder or upper arm may be more safely and conveniently carried out if the patient is intubated as the airway is then secure and the anaesthetist is in less proximity to the surgeon.

The problems associated with hip surgery are principally the problems associated with anaesthesia for the elderly (p. 24). The most common operation is for internal fixation of fractures of the neck of femur due to a fall. There is some evidence to suggest that a spinal block may reduce postoperative morbidity. Early mobility is desirable. Methyl acrylate cement which is used to secure orthopaedic prostheses to bone can cause hypotension which can be limited by preloading of the patient with intravenous fluid. Careful monitoring is essential.

ENDOSCOPIC PROCEDURES

Arthroscopy
See anaesthesia for limb surgery (see above).

Bronchoscopy

Problems
- Hypoxia
- Cardiac dysrhythmias
- Sharing the airway with the surgeon

Local anaesthesia (for the cooperative adult)
1. Spray the palate, pharynx and back of the tongue with a 4% lignocaine solution. Alternatively the patient may suck an amethocaine lozenge.
2. The superior laryngeal nerves are blocked by passing gauze soaked in local anaesthetic over the back of the tongue into the piriform fossae. Special curved forceps (Krause) are used for this purpose.
3. 2 ml of 4% lignocaine is injected through the cricothyroid membrane at the end of a deep expiration. Alternatively the local anaesthetic may be instilled through the glottis, the pharynx and glottis having been previously anaesthetised.

General anaesthesia
Bronchoscopies are normally short procedures and suxamethonium, or mivacurium given by intermittent boluses or an infusion, is used to provide muscular relaxation which allows rapid return of power at completion of the procedure. Maintenance of anaesthesia using an inhalational agent may be difficult and unpleasant for the endoscopist. A total intravenous technique is commonly required. A rapid recovery of consciousness and rapid return of protective reflexes must be an essential part of the technique.

IPPV is provided by the use of a venturi system which injects oxygen down the lumen of the bronchoscope and entrains air through the open end. This technique has revolutionised bronchoscopy under general anaesthesia. Previous methods, which included inserting an endotracheal tube intermittently into the end of the bronchoscope, apnoeic diffusion oxygenation or the simple insufflation of oxygen down the bronchoscope, all resulted in either hypoxia or hypercarbia.

If a fibreoptic bronchoscope is to be used it can either be passed down a rigid bronchoscope, allowing IPPV with the venturi to be continued, or the patient may be intubated and the bronchoscope passed through an air-tight gasket on the connector to the endotracheal tube. Ventilation is maintained using a conventional ventilator.

If a biopsy has been taken the patient should be positioned so that any blood drains away from the 'good' lung and up into the trachea.

Cystoscopy
Many patients have frequent anaesthetics and consideration should be given to the agents used. It has been suggested that halothane should not be repeated within 6 months.

Local anaesthetic techniques are suitable if a general anaesthetic is considered undesirable. Most patients having a cystoscopy will be day-case patients and thus a spinal or epidural may not be the most appropriate chioice. Agents used to provide a general anaesthetic should be chosen to produce a quick recovery and minimal after-effects.

Laparoscopy
Gaseous distension of the abdomen may lead to a reduced venous return, a fall in cardiac output and limitation of diaphragmatic movements. Gas embolism, (see p. 83) and regurgitation are also potential hazards.

Many laparascopic tubal sterilisations are now performed using local anaesthesia in the conscious patient. Tracheal intubation and IPPV is mandatory for general anaesthesia.

Laryngoscopy
See laryngeal surgery, p. 87.

Mediastinoscopy
A mediastinoscope is inserted behind the sternal notch to pass into the upper mediastinum. The potential for serious haemorrhage exists and blood should be immediately available. The trachea should be intubated with an armoured endotracheal tube and IPPV should be instituted. A large-bore peripheral infusion line should be placed.

Oesophagoscopy
Rupture of the oesophagus, damage to the teeth or jaw and regurgitation if oesophageal contents are held above a stricture are all potential hazards. Oesophagoscopy with a flexible instrument may be carried out under sedation. General anaesthesia with intubation of the trachea, full muscular relaxation and IPPV is necessary if a rigid oesophagoscope is to be used. Intermittent suxamethonium or mivacurium are commonly used to provide the muscular relaxation. Intravenous fluid therapy is necessary as it is common practice for the patient to be 'nil by mouth' for 24 hours post-endoscopy.

Ophthalmoscopy
See ophthalmic surgery, p. 85.

RADIOLOGICAL PROCEDURES

NEURORADIOLOGY

The specific problems associated with neurological disease (p. 62) are of obvious importance. The working space is usually cramped, but in addition there are specific problems associated with each procedure.

Cerebral angiography

Problems
- The development of a haematoma in the neck may displace the trachea, leading to partial airway obstruction
- Hypertension or hypotension may occur
- A respiratory arrest may occur if the intracranial pressure is markedly raised
- If the procedure is performed under local anaesthesia a burning sensation on the face and in the retrobulbar region may cause movement with spoiling of the films

Management
- Local anaesthesia with sedation is possible.
- Careful assessment of the required dose of sedative or narcotic is necessary to avoid repiratory depression.

   General anaesthesia using nitrous oxide with a muscle relaxant, intubation with a reinforced tube and IPPV is generally preferred with normocapnia. Hyperventilation reduces the P_aCO_2 and reduces the circulation to normal brain with little effect on the tumour circulation, thus improving the definition of the tumour. On the other hand hyperventilation should be avoided if a subarachnoid haemorrhage is suspected because spasm of blood vessels may be present with a further reduction in blood flow.

Computerised tomography (CT scanning)

Problems
- Monitoring at a distance is required during the procedure.
- Hypoxia, hypercarbia and drugs which increase intracranial pressure should be avoided.

Management
General anaesthesia is required for patients who cannot keep still (e.g. children). An intubation, relaxant, IPPV technique is recommended.

Magnetic resonance imaging (MRI)

Problems
Electrical equipment attached to the patient will disturb the scanning process and the magnet may induce currents in implanted electronic devices (e.g. pacemaker). Leave your credit cards and all metallic objects outside the room.

Management
General anaesthesia is only required for patients who cannot keep still, as for CT scanning.

Non-ferrous connectors must be used. Specially built anaesthetic machines, monitors and connectors constructed from non-magnetic materials are available.

Arterial angiography

Problems
Generalised cardiovascular disease, see p. 42.

Management
For coronary and translumbar aortography a general anaesthetic may be required, and in the case of translumbar aortography IPPV with the patient in the prone position but without the chest and pelvic supports is necessary.

Cardiac catheter studies

Problems
• Those associated with cardiac disease, p. 42
• Increased likelihood of arrhythmias during the positioning of the catheters

Management
General anaesthesia is not usually required for intracardiac pressure and blood gas tension studies. Sedation alone is adequate. For those unable to cooperate, general anaesthesia may be necessary.

The F_1O_2 and P_aCO_2 must be kept constant to allow accurate interpretation of the blood gas tension results. Intrathoracic pressure and cardiac contractility should also be disturbed as little as possible to avoid reversing a shunt, e.g. a left-to-right shunt may be reversed if a rise in intrathoracic pressure leads to a rise in pulmonary artery pressure. Either spontaneous respiration or IPPV may be used. As long as a particular technique is used consistently in one department a reliable interpretation of the results is possible.

PROBLEMS AND TECHNIQUES ASSOCIATED WITH ANAESTHESIA

EFFECTS OF POSTURE

Supine
Muscular relaxation removes the muscle support for the vertebral ligaments, leading to flattening of the lumbar spine with postoperative backache. The supine hypotensive syndrome is associated with patients with an intra-abdominal mass, e.g. pregnancy.

Prone
Anterior/posterior expansion of the chest is reduced and diaphragm movements are reduced if the patient is not supported off the table to allow abdominal expansion. Pillows under the chest and pelvis are commonly used.

Lateral
Gravity reduces the blood flow to the upper lung. During IPPV pressure of the abdominal contents on the dependent hemidiaphragm reduces expansion of the lower lung. Ventilation and perfusion of the lungs is therefore mismatched. During spontaneous respiration the dependent diaphragm is elevated, because of the pressure of the abdominal contents, and therefore when it contracts it sweeps out a larger volume than the upper diaphragm. Ventilation and perfusion are more equally matched. If the chest is opened, mediastinal shift may occur with deleterious consequences; flow through the inferior vena cava is reduced and therefore the cardiac output falls.

Lithotomy
There is a marked reduction in the vital capacity. Damage to the hip and vertebral joints is possible, particulary if they have limited movement.

Trendelenburg
The head-down position results in diaphragmatic splinting and, in the susceptible patient, promotes regurgitation of gastric contents. The airway and ventilation must be protected. The central blood volume is increased.

Reverse Trendelenburg
The head-up tilt decreases the central blood volume due to the pooling of blood in the legs. This posture, on its own or in conjunction with depressant drugs, may cause hypotension. Venous ooze is reduced in the elevated parts of the body.

Parry Brown
This position has been used to facilitate the drainage of secretions from the tracheobronchial tree during thoracic surgery. The patient lies prone with the hips elevated above the level of the shoulders and the head turned to the side of the operation. The arm on the operative side hangs down by the side of the table. On opening the chest there is no mediastinal shift.

Nerve damage
Nerve damage can occur in many positions. The commonest are from excessive abduction of the arms and depression of the shoulders (brachial plexus), pressure on the outside aspect of lower legs against lithotomy poles (lateral popliteal), and compression of the upper arm (radial nerve). In addition, ischaemic damage may result from undue pressure on any vulnerable part, e.g. nose, ear.

CANNULATION OF VESSELS

Peripheral veins
Avoid sites close to joints, infusions in the legs (increased incidence of thrombophlebitis or thrombosis), and irritant fluids. A central venous cannula should preferably be used for such fluids. Cannulas should be changed 24-hourly or, more realistically, at the first sign of any tissue reaction.

Central veins

Antecubital fossa
The antecubital fossa can be used for the insertion of central venous catheters and either the basilic or cephalic vein may be cannulated. The course of the cephalic vein passes through the clavipectoral fascia and it is at this point that the cannula may be held up. The basilic vein passes more deeply, becoming the axillary vein, and passage of the catheter is less likely to be impeded. An X-ray must be taken to confirm the position of the tip of the catheter.

Subclavian
The subclavian vein passes over the first rib and then medially and downwards. Its highest point is just medial to the midpoint of the clavicle. To cannulate this vessel the patient should be supine with the head turned away from the site of insertion. Head-down tilt is desirable—this fills the vein and minimises the risk of air embolism. The cannula is inserted 1 cm below the lower border of the clavicle and just lateral to its midpoint. It is directed to pass just below the clavicle towards the suprasternal notch. On the left side the thoracic duct may be damaged. X-ray confirmation of position is desirable before use.

Internal jugular
At its lower end the internal jugular vein is covered by the sternomastoid muscle. With the patient supine, head-down, and with the head turned away from the site of injection, the cannula is inserted 3 cm above the clavicle and just lateral to the lateral border of the sternomastoid, the needle being directed towards the supra-sternal notch. X-ray confirmation of position is desirable.

External jugular
The external jugular vein is superficial and crosses the sternomastoid muscle. It is relatively easy to cannulate but it may be difficult to get the cannula to pass into the subclavian vein.

Femoral
The femoral vein lies medial to the femoral artery, which is found at the midpoint between the anterior superior iliac spine and the pubic symphysis. With a catheter of sufficient length central venous pressures can be measured.

Uses include measurement of central venous pressure or passage of a pulmonary artery flotation (Swan–Ganz) catheter, parenteral nutrition, infusion of hyperosmolar or vasoactive agents, haemodialysis or haemofiltration.

Complications
The complications of central venous cannulation include infection, haematoma, pneumothorax, hydrothorax, haemothorax and cardiac tamponade (due to perforation of the atrial wall by the cannula). It is also possible to create an arterio-venous fistula.

Arteries

Brachial artery
The brachial artery crosses the elbow joint anteriorly. Its anatomy is variable and it can be considered an end artery as its occlusion can result in distal ischaemia if the collateral circulation is insufficient. It is superficial, being covered only by skin and fascia, and cannulation is not difficult.

Radial artery
This artery runs lateral to the tendon of flexor carpi ulnaris at the wrist. Before cannulation of this artery Allen's test should be carried out to establish patency of the ulnar artery. The hand is exsanguinated following compression of both radial artery and ulnar artery. Release of the pressure over the ulnar artery should result in a flushing of the hand if circulation via the ulnar artery is adequate.

Femoral artery
The femoral artery passes deep to the inguinal ligament, midway between the anterior superior iliac spine and the pubic symphysis. The vein lies medial and the nerve lateral to the artery.

Dorsalis pedis
The dorsalis pedis artery is on the dorsum of the foot between the tendons of extensor hallucis longus and extensor digitorum longus, at the root of the cleft between the first and second toes. A modified Allen's test should be performed on the foot with occlusion of the dorsalis pedis and the posterior tibial arteries.

Cannulation techniques
The general technique for cannulation of arteries is:
1. Test for adequacy of collateral circulation.
2. Raise a weal of local anaesthetic if the patient is conscious.
3. Palpate and fix artery by skin tension or by straddling the artery with fingers.
4. Enter the artery directly using either a needle through catheter or a needle and guidewire set.
5. Secure the line carefully and label the line such that it cannot be confused with an intravenous line and inadvertently used for drug administration.

Uses
• Pressure monitoring and blood sampling

Complications
• Ischaemia in the distal tissues supplied by the artery
• Haemorrhage
• Nerve damage if artery and nerve adjacent

CONTROL OF P_aCO_2 DURING ANAESTHESIA

Hypocapnia
• Sympathetic tone is reduced
• Cardiac output is decreased
• Peripheral vasoconstriction develops
• The pain threshold is raised with a decrease in MAC values, resulting in a reduction of drug dosage
• Postoperative respiratory depression is possible

Normocapnia
• Sympathetic tone is not changed
• Cardiac output is maintained
• Postoperative respiratory depression is unlikely
• Greater doses of drugs are required to maintain the patient pain-free and the muscles relaxed

Hypercapnia
• Sympathetic tone is reduced with peripheral vasodilation
• Risk of cardiac arrhythmias is increased
• In general, hypercapnia should be avoided

NASO-GASTRIC INTUBATION

Naso-gastric intubation is carried out to facilitate aspiration of gastric secretions, to detect and monitor gastric and small bowel stasis, or for feeding. Naso-gastric intubation should only be carried out if it is necessary, as it has disadvantages. The incidence of chest infections is increased, the integrity of the cardiac sphincter impaired and the pharynx irritated. Incorrect positioning can result in instillation of fluids into the lungs with potentially fatal results. Its position should be verified before use. For details of naso-gastric feeding regimens see p. 166.

PULMONARY ASPIRATION SYNDROME

The inhalation of gastric contents is associated with a high morbidity and mortality. Its occurrence in obstetric anaesthetic practice is termed 'Mendelson's syndrome' and has a high mortality rate, although when it was originally described (1946) it did not. Factor(s) involved in modern anaesthetic or obstetric practice have therefore altered the picture of the condition.

The effects of acid in the lungs include inflammation, exudation and the production of haemorrhagic oedema fluid. Hyaline membranes occur and there is destruction of lung parenchyma. The pH of the acid has to be below 2.5 to produce this picture in experimental animals.

Factors which increase the risk of regurgitation should always be noted and attempts made to minimise the risk. Active emptying of the stomach either by the passage of a wide-bore stomach tube or by the use of an emetic has been advocated. Head-up tilt, if the situation allows, will minimise passive movement of gastric contents up the oesophagus and thence into the airway. The prophylactic use of antacids is now routine in obstetric anaesthesia. Protection of the airway by endotracheal intubation is mandatory if the patient is at risk and the rapid sequence induction techniques with cricoid pressure should be followed (p. 82).

Management of the pulmonary aspiration syndrome
1. The airway should be cleared of gross contaminants by head-down tilt and suction. Bronchoscopy may be necessary. Oxygenation should be maintained and intubation is desirable.
2. Bronchial lavage is carried out in an attempt to reduce further chemical irritation by the inhaled acidic fluid. Normal saline is probably the best solution to use. Dilute sodium bicarbonate solution has been used in an attempt to neutralise the acid but is itself irritant.
3. Steroids are given for their anti-inflammatory effect; bronchospasm may also be reduced.

4. Specific agents may be required for the treatment of bronchospasm—e.g. adrenaline, aminophylline, salbutomal and atropine.
5. Respiratory failure may ensue and IPPV may be required.

ONE-LUNG ANAESTHESIA

One-lung anaesthesia may inadvertently be used if a single-lumen endotracheal tube slips down one (usually the right) main bronchus. Following intubation, chest movements and air entry should be checked to ensure that this situation does not exist or persist.

One-lung anaesthesia is electively used during intrathoracic procedures where the inflated lung would impede surgical access or where there is a large air leak from one lung making effective ventilation difficult. Many endobronchial tubes have been designed for the purpose but the most common double-lumen endobronchial tube in use today is the Robertshaw. It is designed so that it is easy to position and the internal cross-sectional area is maximised, thus reducing the resistance to ventilation and facilitating the passage of a suction catheter for aspiration of secretions.

The effects of ventilating one lung and collapsing the other vary from one patient to another. The greatest physiological change occurs in those patients with normal lungs as the passage of a large proportion of the cardiac output through an unventilated lung results in systemic hypoxia. The patient who has had a partly occluded main bronchus for some time, due to neoplasia, will show little change.

Shunts of between 20% and 65% of the cardiac output may result from the passage of blood through the unventilated lung. Hypoxia can be reduced but not prevented by increasing the inspired concentration of oxygen, thus maximising the oxygenation of blood passing through the ventilated lung. Reduction in tidal volume and an increase in frequency of ventilation may be required to maintain minute volume but at the same time keep the airway pressure within the acceptable range. Venous return to the heart is reduced due to the exposure of the mediastinal veins to atmospheric pressure. If mediastinal shift occurs, and the great veins become kinked, then a catastrophic fall in cardiac output may result.

On reinflation of the lung all segments must be checked to ensure full aeration. Postoperataive atelectasis may be a problem. A short period of elective controlled ventilation with positive end-expiratory pressure may be required.

INDUCED HYPOTENSION DURING ANAESTHESIA

An improved surgical field may be produced by the use of a tourniquet on an exsanguinated limb, by the use of local vasonstrictor agents or by the use of induced hypotension. The major hazard of induced hypotension is cerebral ischaemia and thus the indication for hypotension is the virtual impossibility of surgery without a bloodless field. The benefits must outweigh the risks. Certain patients are more clearly at risk, e.g. those with a past history of cerebral ischaemia and those with an existing oxygen transport problem.

General principles

1. Continous cardiovascular monitoring is essential and cerebral function monitoring is ideal as it is impossible to predict the adequacy of cerebral perfusion in advance. IPPV is usually employed during induced hypotension as the physiological dead space may be reduced; however, spontaneous respiration is used by some as a means of monitoring medullary perfusion.
2. The practice of good general anaesthesia minimises the need for specific hypotensive agents:
   a. No venous congestion due to respiratory obstruction or coughing
   b. Reduced sympathetic tone by adequate oxygenation, ventilation and analgesia
3. Posture. If possible the operative site should be positioned uppermost to enhance venous drainage. The monitoring of pressure must take into account the pressure difference (vertical height) between the site of measurement and the brain.
4. Drugs such as halothane that produce myocardial depression and/or vasodilatation are commonly employed. A reduction in cardiac output, however, is not desirable.
5. Ganglionic blockade, either by specific agents or by agents that have this action as a side-effect, is also used. Spinal and epidural anaesthesia fall into the latter group; trimetaphan into the former.
6. Sodium nitroprusside has specific action on vascular smooth muscle and when administered as an infusion produces a controllable fall in peripheral resistance, arterial blood pressure and central venous pressure. Heart rate and cardiac output rise. Care must be taken not to administer a toxic dose in either total amount given or in the rate. The antidote, sodium nitrite and vitamin B_{12a}, must be available.
7. If a compensatory tachycardia negates the effect of the hypotensive agent being used then a beta-2 adrenergic receptor blocker may be used (take care in patients prone to bronchospasm). Other causes of tachycardia should be excluded.

At the conclusion of the procedure the blood pressure should be allowed to rise slowly, haemostasis should be secured and blood loss should be replaced. Good postoperative care with pain relief and oxygen by mask are essential.

CONTROL OF INTRAVENOUS DRUG CONCENTRATIONS

The physicochemical properties of a drug, the degree of protein binding, the regional distribution of blood flow and in some instances active transport mechanisms determine to which of the variety of 'compartments' within the body the drug is distributed. Drug distribution may be confined to anatomical compartments; for example, heparin is confined to the plasma water.

The volume of distribution, a purely mathematical concept, is expressed as

$$V_D = \frac{X}{C}$$

where X is total amount of drug and C is plasma concentration. The volume of distribution affects drug concentration and also influences drug action. If the pharmacokinetics of a particular drug's distribution are known, the administration may be planned to maintain a near-constant circulatory concentration. Multicompartmental computer models have been constructed to improve the control of drug administration and hence the predictability of their effects.

In clinical practice a loading dose of the drug is usually given followed by a constant infusion if rapid achievement of the desired concentration/effect is necessary. The infusion rate is then adjusted according to the patient's response.

TARGET-CONTROLLED INFUSION

This new concept uses an infusion pump into which is programmed the pharmacokinetics of a drug, based on the population mean. The operator, instead of selecting the infusion rate, selects the desired plasma concentration. The microprocessor in the pump then delivers a bolus followed by an exponentially declining infusion rate to reach and maintain the desired plasma concentration without further operator intervention. The system is presently only available for propofol.

RESPIRATORY PHYSIOTHERAPY

Breathing exercises in the preoperative period may be used to increase the vital capacity by encouraging diaphragmatic movements and effective coughing. Postural drainage of diseased segments or normal areas of the lungs allows secretions to collect in the main bronchi. These may then be cleared by coughing.

For those patients who require IPPV, application of vibratory movements to the chest wall, postural drainage and associated pulmonary expansion by squeezing of a reservoir bag has proved effective in maintaining good pulmonary ventilation and preventing atelectasis.

DEEP VEIN THROMBOSIS PROPHYLAXIS

Deep vein thrombosis frequently occurs in the veins of the calf, although other parts of the peripheral venous system, e.g. pelvic veins, may also be involved. Immobility during prolonged surgery or during the postoperative period may lead to venous stasis which may, particularly when associated with dehydration and altered blood coagulability, promote deep vein thrombosis.

Diagnosis may be made on clinical evidence, e.g. oedema, swelling, redness and tenderness in the calf, but is confirmed using either the Doppler ultrasound technique or the uptake of ^{125}T-labelled fibrinogen. The serious hazard is potentially fatal pulmonary embolism associated with severe chest pain, dyspnoea and right ventricular failure.

Venous stasis may be reduced by hydration and the use of physiotherapy, elastic stockings, leg elevation and intermittent compression of the calf muscles by pneumatic leggings. In high-risk patients, prophylactic measures must be continued throughout the period of risk until the patient is fully ambulant. High-risk patients are those who have a past history of venous thromboembolism, immobility (e.g. plaster of Paris cast) and those who are patients undergoing abdominal or pelvic surgery for malignant disease. One-third of these patients may develop a deep venous thrombosis; 2% may suffer a fatal pulmonary embolism. Many other factors predispose to thrombus formation: age, obesity, varicose veins and infection. Early postoperative mobilisation is essential.

External pneumatic compression of the calves may be used in conjunction with any of the other prophylactic measures. The prophylactic use of subcutaneous or low molecular weight heparin and oral anticoagulation have been shown to be of value. An effective regime is 5000 units of heparin 2 hours preoperatively and 8 hours postoperatively, but this has a slightly increased risk of wound haematoma. Oral anticoagulation to double the prothrombin time reduces thrombus formation but increases the risk of bleeding to an unacceptable level. A lesser degree of anticoagulation reduces this risk but does not prevent thrombi forming, although it may reduce thromboembolism.

CHEST DRAINS

The function of a chest drain is to allow gas or fluid to leave the pleural space and at the same time prevent the ingress of air. The commonly used sites for the insertion of a chest drain are the anterior axillary line in the second intercostal space and the mid axillary line in the fifth intercostal space. The latter is more comfortable for the patient and the resulting scar is in a less noticeable position. Damage to vessels and nerves is avoided if the trocar is inserted immediately above the lower rib as the nerves and vessels lie beneath the inferior border of the ribs. Large intrathoracic vessels are less likely to be damaged if the 1–2 cm of intercostal space just lateral to the sternum is avoided.

Following pneumonectomy a chest drain may be inserted to allow assessment of postoperative bleeding. It is normally clamped off and only released intermittently to assess the loss. In this situation the chest drain may also be used to adjust the position of the mediastinum if a shift has occurred—air may be allowed into the space or removed from it as the situation dictates.

Following a lobectomy or similar procedure where lung tissue remains in the hemithorax, chest drains are used to evacuate the pleural space of air which encourages the inflation of the lung. They may be connected to a low-pressure vacuum pump for this purpose (up to 10 cm H_2O vacuum). If the chest drain has been inserted as a treatment for a tension pneumothorax then it should under no circumstances be clamped or attached to a vacuum pump. The flow of gas through the chest drain may exceed the capacity of the pump and thus the pump will retard the drainage of the gas and a tension pneumothorax may recur.

DEFIBRILLATION

Defibrillation is the passage of an electrical current across the heart to terminate ventricular fibrillation (VF) or to convert atrial or ventricular tachyarrythmias to a normal rhythm. Defibrillators can deliver up to 400 joules. Large-diameter paddle electrodes are used to prevent burns.

Ventricular fibrillation
The defibrillation energy stops the chaotic electrical activity and, by synchronising the refractory periods of the muscle fibres, allows the pacemaker to regain control. The shock can be given at any time as there is no organised activity.

Ventricular or atrial tachyarrythmias
Depolarisation of the whole heart during the refractory period allows the sino-atrial node to regain control. A synchronised shock has to be given during cardioversion or VF may result from the electrical pulse coinciding with a T-wave—the vulnerable period during the electromechanical cycle. The R-wave is used to trigger the defibrillator.

The maximum energy (360–400 joules) is often required when treating VF, but when a cardioversion is being carried out, a lower level of energy is used (start at 20 joules) and this is increased stepwise as necessary. Electrode jelly must not be allowed to run between the paddles, and personnel must keep clear of the bed, the patient and all attached lines during the administration of the shock.

MASSIVE BLOOD TRANSFUSION

The transfusion of large quantities of blood (more than about 15 litres) is associated with a high morbidity, although in certain patients, transfusion of quantities less than this may also produce similar problems. Many of these problems can be anticipated and corrective measures taken.

1. Accurate cross-matching of the blood will minimise the probability of a transfusion reaction.
2. Filtering of blood will remove much of the debris that accumulates in stored blood and will prevent the lungs from becoming loaded with this particulate matter.
3. Warming the blood will reduce the likelihood of hypothermia secondary to the infusion of several litres of fluid at 4°C. The temperature of the heating device should not exceed 42°C.
4. A dilutional coagulopathy should be anticipated and a clotting screen should be obtained early in the procedure. If it is normal it will act as a baseline for later results. Platelets and fresh frozen plasma will be required.
5. The potassium and calcium equilibrium may be disturbed but there is little evidence that active measures are required. Citrate toxicity is unlikely unless the metabolic state of the patient is severely impaired—liver failure, hypothermia and renal failure.
6. Stored blood is acidic (pH around 6.5) and the administration of bicarbonate has been suggested. This is no longer recommended as a routine unless blood gas analysis has been carried out and the acid/base state requires to be urgently corrected. In the longer term, citrate will be metabolised and result in a metabolic alkalosis.
7. The problems that are encountered in all transfusions are accentuated when the volumes to be infused are increased—air embolism, infection, transmission of disease and circulatory embarrassment.

Anticipation of the above problems and an accurate assessment of the blood loss, together with careful monitoring of the circulatory state should result in a patient who has an adequate circulatory volume, an adequate state of perfusion and adequate oxygen transport.

TRACHEOTOMY

A tracheotomy is carried out by extending the head, without rotation, and making a midline incision. The large vessels in the neck are pushed back with the fingers, to behind the sternomastoid muscles. Retraction of the thyroid isthmus upwards will enable palpation of the trachea. Two or three tracheal rings are incised, 2nd, 3rd and/or 4th and the sides of the incision are held apart until a tube is inserted. A stitch may be placed on each side of the incision to hold the sides apart. Incision of the first tracheal ring should be avoided because it may lead to subsequent tracheal stenosis and an incision that is too low may endanger the innominate vessels. This procedure should only be performed as an emergency life-saving measure. A percutaneous dilatational tracheostomy or surgical tracheostomy should normally be the technique of choice.

HEPATITIS INFECTION PRECAUTIONS

Accidental infection with the virus of serum hepatitis (B or C especially) can result in serious liver damage or death. High-risk patients are those who are known to be positive on testing for the hepatitis B or C antigen or antibody, those patients requiring regular haemodialysis, drug addicts and those jaundiced patients in whom a diagnosis has yet to be made.

To prevent contamination of the skin, eyes, nose and mouth it is suggested that all personnel should be gowned and masked, and goggles and gloves should be worn. Venepuncture should be carried out with disposable equipment. Spilt blood or body fluids should be diluted with strong hypochlorite solution and wiped up with a disposable cloth. Disposable items should be used whenever possible and all disposable items should be placed in a plastic bag which should be sealed and labelled correctly for subsequent incineration.

4. Local anaesthetic techniques, postoperative analgesia and the management of chronic pain

LOCAL ANAESTHETIC TECHNIQUES

GENERAL APPROACH

1. Examine the patient for
   a. Sepsis
   b. CNS/Spinal disorders
   c. Skeletal abnormalities/surface landmarks
   d. Evidence of a bleeding diathesis or anticoagulant therapy
2. Exclude allergy and anticoagulant therapy
3. Explain to the patient the nature of the procedure
4. Check resuscitation equipment
5. Insert intravenous cannula
6. Position patient
   a. Prepare site(s) of injection
   b. Check equipment, needles, catheters, ampoules, etc.
7. Perform block
8. Observe patient for any untoward effects, drowsiness, tinnitus and numbness of lips and tongue, indicative of toxic concentrations of local anaesthetic. Tremors and convulsions are late signs of toxicity. True allergy to local anaesthetic agents is extremely rare. The signs of CNS toxicity are usually, incorrectly, described as 'allergy'.

NERVE BLOCKS FOR SURGERY OF THE HEAD AND NECK

SCALP AND CRANIUM

A band of infiltration from glabella, above ear, to occiput blocks all nerves. Inject three layers—skin, subcutaneous tissue and periosteum if bone is to be removed. The temporalis muscle may need to be infiltrated.

EYE

1. Infiltration of eyelids
2. Retrobulbar injection within muscle cone (ciliary nerve and ganglion are blocked)

3. Block facial nerve at neck of mandible, just below the zygoma (prevent squeezing of the eyeball by orbicularis oculi)

The retrobulbar block may be performed by a superior approach (Macintosh) through the superior rectus with the patient looking down, or by the infero-lateral approach (Atkinson) from a point at the infero-lateral margin of the orbit passing backwards along the floor of the orbit.

NOSE

Parts of both the I and II divisions of the trigeminal nerve (V) innervate the nose:

Ophthalmic N (I)   Supratrochlear branch of frontal
                    anterior ethmoidal branch of nasociliary
Maxillary N (II)   Infra-orbital branch
                    Long sphenopalatine (sphenopalatine ganglion)

- Frontal nerve: inject 1 cm above caruncle; proceed laterally to roof of orbit.
- Anterior ethmoidal nerve: inject 1 cm above caruncle, 3.5 cm along wall of orbit.
- Infra-orbital branch: inject 1 cm below orbital margin, directly below pupil.
- Sphenopalatine ganglion: inject 0.5 cm below midpoint of zygoma, interior to the coronoid. At a depth of 4 cm the lateral pterygoid plate is encountered; advance 1 cm anteriorly into the pterygo-maxillary fissure. Withdraw plunger before injection as the orbit or pharynx may have been entered.

THROAT

A tonsil block involves the lesser palatine branch of the maxillary nerve (II division of V) and the lingual branch of the mandibular nerve (III division of V). A glossopharyngeal nerve (IX) block is also necessary.
Technique: a local anaesthetic lozenge is sucked and later the upper parts of the anterior and posterior pillars, and the infra- and supratonsillar areas are infiltrated.

The larynx (Fig. 4.1) and pharynx

Sensory	Mucous membrane above cords and below epiglottis	VAGUS N	Internal laryngeal N
	Mucous membrane below oropharynx, posterior 1/3 tongue	VAGUS N	Recurrent laryngeal N
	Superior surface of epiglottis	GLOSSOPHARYNGEAL N	
	Nasopharynx	SPHENOPALATINE N	

Motor	Cricothyroid, inferior constrictor	VAGUS N	External laryngeal N
	Intrinsic muscles of larynx	VAGUS N	Recurrent laryngeal N
	Pharynx and palate	VAGUS N	Pharyngeal plexus

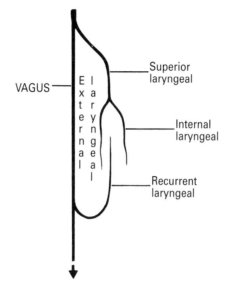

Fig 4.1   The laryngeal nerves

Vagus nerve block—technique

The patient lies supine and looks straight ahead. The pinna is held forward. A needle is inserted just anterior to the tip of the mastoid process, angled 30° anteriorly. At a depth of 4 cm an aspiration test is carried out and then 2 ml of local anaesthetic is injected, the needle is withdrawn 0.5 cm and a further injection made. Veins, arteries and nasopharynx may all be punctured and the superior cervical sympathetic ganglion, glossopharyngeal, accessory and hypoglossal nerves may all be affected. Airway obstruction can result.

Mandibular nerve blocks for dental surgery

The mandibular nerve is division III of the Vth cranial nerve.

Extra-oral approach

The mouth is opened wide and the position of the condyle marked; the needle is inserted at this point, horizontally and slightly anteriorly. At 4 cm the lateral pterygoid plate is encountered. Position a marker 0.5 cm from the skin and redirect the needle posteriorly. Inject 2 ml of local anaesthetic and 5 ml more as the needle is withdrawn.

Intra-oral approach
Using the index finger, placed lateral to the lower molars, palpate the anterior edge of the ramus of the mandible. Rotate the finger into the retromolar fossa and advance the finger to touch the internal oblique ridge. The needle is inserted 0.1 to 1 cm medial to the midline of the fingernail and lateral to the pterygomandibular ligament. As soon as the buccinator is pierced (lingual and long buccal nerves are blocked), 0.5 ml of local anaesthetic is injected; advance the needle a further 2.5 cm and inject a further 2 ml. This will block the inferior dental nerve.

Cervical plexus blocks for surgery of the neck (Fig. 4.2)
Nerves C2, C3 and C4 lie in the groove between the anterior and posterior tubercles of the transverse processes of the respective cervical vertebrae and lie therefore in the plane which exists between the muscles originating from these tubercles. The transverse process of C3 lies behind the carotid artery at the level of the hyoid bone. With the patient looking slightly to the opposite side the carotid sheath is displaced medially and a needle inserted to just pass through the edge of sternocleidomastoid, backwards and medially until the bone is reached. The needle should be passed beyond the transverse process so that infiltration is ensured on withdrawal. Then 5 ml of local anaesthetic is injected. C2 and C4 are blocked through the same point of entry through the skin. The phrenic and vagus nerves and sympathetic chain may all be involved.

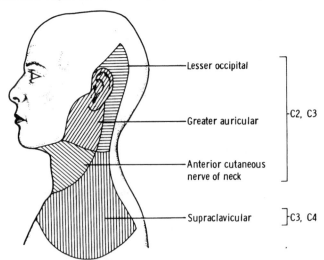

Fig 4.2 Sensory dermatomes served by C2, C3, C4

Sympathetic blockade

Stellate ganglion
Vascular insufficiency of the upper limbs, pulmonary embolism, post-thoracotomy pain, status asthmaticus, angina, herpes zoster are some of the indications suggested for a stellate ganglion block.

Paratracheal approach (Moore)
With the patient lying supine the head is extended without a pillow and the needle is inserted 3 cm lateral to, and above, the jugular notch. Advance the needle posteriorly; when the transverse process of C7 is touched, withdraw 0.5 cm and inject 10 ml of local anaesthetic.

Sweating, salivation and bronchial secretions are reduced by the block. Vasodilation occurs and cardiac pain is abolished. Horner's syndrome results, miosis, enophthalmos and ptosis; and intraocular pressure falls.

Complication are numerous—the phrenic nerve and brachial plexus may be blocked and intrathecal and epidural injections may also be made. Pneumothorax, oesophageal puncture, intravascular injection (vertebral artery), block of cardio-accelerator fibres (sympathetic ganglia), hoarseness (recurrent laryngeal nerve block) have been reported.

NERVE BLOCKS FOR SURGERY OF THE TRUNK, PERINEUM AND LEGS

- Epidural
- Spinal
- Paravertebral   Anatomy and physiology—see pp. 144–146
- Intercostal
- Autonomic blocks

Epidural block (Fig. 4.3)

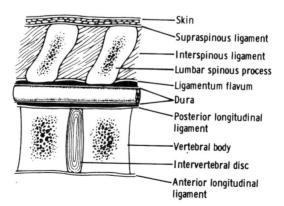

Skin
Supraspinous ligament
Interspinous ligament
Lumbar spinous process
Ligamentum flavum
Dura
Posterior longitudinal ligament
Vertebral body
Intervertebral disc
Anterior longitudinal ligament

Fig 4.3   Sagittal section through the lumbar spine

Contraindications
- Sepsis
- Haemorrhagic diathesis, anticoagulant therapy
- Acute or chronic disease of the CNS
- Neurological disease (e.g. multiple sclerosis)
- Raised intracranial pressure

Complications	*Treatment*
Headache	1. Increase fluid intake
	2. Blood patch
Hypotension	Fluids, posture, vasopressor
Patchy analgesia	A larger volume of injectate may overcame the inadequate block
Respiratory depression (too high a block)	Positive pressure ventilation
Convulsions	Positive pressure ventilation, muscle relaxation, anticonvulsants
Urinary retention	Catheterisation
Spinal subarachnoid puncture	See below
Epidural abscess or haematoma	Surgical decompression
Spinal artery thrombosis	
Spinal cord or nerve root damage	
Aseptic or septic meningitis	
Arachnoiditis	
Backache	

Lumbar epidural technique
The patient is placed in the lateral position with the hips, knees and neck flexed. The back must be perpendicular to the floor and the lumbar spine parallel to edge of the bed.

Infiltrate the intervertebral space—subcutaneously and then more deeply into the interspinous space. Perforate the skin with a large-bore needle. Insert and advance the epidural needle until the epidural space is located. Confirmation of the needle position may be achieved by either a loss-of-resistance technique or by a change in electrical conductivity that occurs on entering the space.

Loss of resistance
- Syringe with air or saline
- Macintosh balloon
- Odom's indicator
- Hanging drop method

Local anaesthetic, 10–20 ml, is injected in a 'single shot' or a catheter is inserted 2–3 cm beyond the tip of the needle, the needle withdrawn, a bacterial filter attached and then the local anaesthetic is injected. During late pregnancy use only 2/3 of the normal dose, as the spread of the local anaesthetic is increased. Reduce the dose in the elderly.

Problems
Identification of the space—obesity, calcification of ligaments, poor flexion. Dural puncture with loss of CSF—perform the epidural in another space. Physiological saline is infused into the space through a catheter for 24 hours to minimise the leakage of CSF by raising the pressure in the epidural space. General hydration must also be maintained. 'Low pressure' headache may last up to a week.

Blood patches have been used in an attempt to seal the hole; however, their use must be weighed against the possible danger of providing a nidus for infection.

Blood-stained tap—try another space up or down.

Thoracic epidural
A thoracic epidural has contraindications, complications and difficulties comparable with those which may follow a lumbar epidural. In addition, the vertebral spines are closer together and angled caudally. A lateral approach may be easier than the conventional midline approach used in the lumbar region.

Insert a neddle 1 cm lateral to the caudal end of the spinous process and infiltrate to the vertebral arch. The epidural needle is inserted and advanced in the same direction but allowed to pass above the arch into the interlaminar space. Further advancement of the needle is made whilst testing for loss of resistance.

Success of the lateral technique depends less on spinal flexion, avoids calcified ligaments, and allows easy passage of the epidural catheter.

Spinal subarachnoid block (Fig. 4.4)
• Contraindications–as for epidural
• Position–lateral or sitting

Technique
A fine-bore pencil point needle (25–27 G) is passed through a guide (a Sise introducer), and advanced until CSF is seen in the lumen.

The height of local anaesthetic spread is limited by specific gravity, posture (degree of head-up or head-down tilt), spinal curvature, the volume and rate of the injection and barbotage. Hypo and isobaric solutions are not now used because of the dangers of a high spinal. The site of action of drug injected at L3, the highest point of the lumbar curve, can be affected by posture. Noradrenaline added to the local anaesthetic may cause ischaemia of the spinal cord.

T5–6 is the lowest point of the thoracic curve and local anaesthetic 'pooled' here can be used to provide a spinal anaesthetic for upper abdominal surgery. At this level the block will also interrupt the sympathetic supply to the viscera.

Hyperbaric bupivacaine is the agent most commonly used in a volume of 2–3 ml. The larger the volume, the higher the block in general.

The lumbar region is used for spinal anaesthesia because there is less possibility of damage to the spinal cord, which in the adult ends at the L1/2 level. For 'mid' and 'low' spinals the sitting position is favoured because flexion is more easily obtained, CSF pressure is higher and the dorsal midline is not distorted by sagging skin.

L3   T6 T5

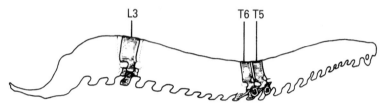

Fig 4.4 Spinal curves indicating highest and lowest points when the patient is supine

Complications
- Dry tap
- Blood-stained tap—if the CSF remains blood-stained the procedure may have to be abandoned
- Hypotension—posture, fluids and vasoconstrictor (ephedrine)
- Total spinal—maintain ventilation and treat hypotension as above
- Headache—the smaller the needle the less likely it is that low-pressure headaches will occur; treat symptomatically and maintain hydration. The rapid infusion of crystalloid solution, 500 ml, can reduce headache. Consider blood patch.

Paravertebral block (Fig. 4.5)
The paravertebral space is wedge-shaped. It communicates laterally with the intercostal space and medially with the epidural space. It is limited anteriorly by the parietal pleura and posteriorly by the costotransverse ligament.

Thoracic—weals are raised 3 cm from the midline opposite the lower borders of the spines. The needle is inserted perpendicular to the skin until contact is made with the transverse process. The needle is then directed over the upper border of the transverse process and the local anaesthetic, 5–10 ml, injected.

Lumbar—the weals are raised opposite the upper border of the spines.

Intercostal nerve blocks (Fig. 4.6)
Spinal level:	Region of anaesthesia:
T2–T6	From sternal angle to xiphisternum
T7–T9	From xiphisternum to umbilicus
T10	Umbilicus
T11-L1	From umbilicus to pubis

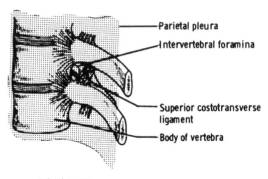

Parietal pleura
Intervertebral foramina
Superior costotransverse ligament
Body of vertebra

Fig 4.5 The paravertebral space

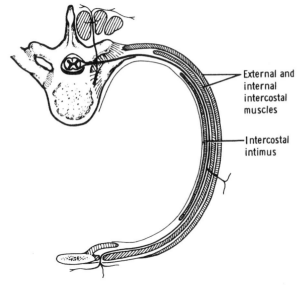

External and internal intercostal muscles
Intercostal intimus

Fig 4.6 The course of the intercostal nerves

Approaches
1. At the angle of the ribs
2. Posterior axillary line
   a. The angle of the ribs is located at the lateral margin of the erector spinae muscles. The patient is placed in the lateral position and two lines are drawn: 7–8 cm from the midline, from scapulae to iliac crests. A needle is inserted at points where the ribs cross the lines and is then advanced until contact is made with the rib. It is then withdrawn slightly and redirected below the lower edge of the rib; 2–3 ml of local anaesthetic is injected.

b. The posterior axillary line approach is similar to that described above except that the posterior axillary line is the longitudinal surface marking. Using this approach the lateral cutaneous nerves are not included within the block.

Autonomic blocks
- Thoracic
- Lumbar
- Coeliac plexus

1. Thoracic sympathetic blockade may be indicated for biliary and renal colic, acute pancreatitis, angina or asthma. The ganglia lie on the heads of the ribs covered by costal pleura.

   Weals are raised 3 cm from the midline over the transverse processes of the desired vertebrae. The needles are inserted so as to impinge on the transverse process and then slipped inferior to them. A marker is set at 4 cm and the needle advanced in a medial direction. An aspiration test is carried out and 5 ml of local anaesthetic is injected.
2. Lumbar sympathetic block may be indicated for peripheral artery disease, traumatic vasospasm and acute arterial occlusion. The ganglia lie on the anterolateral aspects of the lumbar vertebral bodies.

   Mandl's posterior approach is performed in the lateral position with the spine flexed. Weals, 5 cm lateral to the upper borders of the spinous processes of L2, L3 and L4, are raised. Insert needle perpendicularly for 4–5 cm onto the transverse process and then direct upwards and inwards 3–4 cm. Aspirate and then inject local anaesthetic.
3. Coeliac plexus block is normally performed for the relief of pain originating in the upper abdomen as a result of malignant disease. Use X-ray control.

Technique—Kappis method
Identify the first lumbar spine and raise a weal 7–8 cm lateral to it—below the 12th rib. Insert a long needle at an angle of 45° to the median plane and in a slightly upward direction. Contact should be made with the body of L1. Redirect slightly laterally and glance past the body, advance the needle 1 cm more, aspirate and inject 20–40 ml of local anaesthetic. Hypotension is controlled, if necessary, by intravenous fluid infusion or by a vasopressor.

SPECIFIC NERVE BLOCKS FOR PERINEAL SURGERY
- Saddle block
- Caudal
- Pudendal
- Paracervical

SADDLE BLOCK

The spread of a spinal subarachnoid anaesthetic block may be restricted by a dose and posture such that only the saddle area is affected. A hyperbaric local anaesthetic solution is used with the patient in the sitting position.

CAUDAL BLOCK

A caudal block is a form of epidural anaesthesia. Local anaesthetic is injected into the epidural space via the sacral hiatus—to block T10–T12 a large volume is required. Dural puncture is rare, as the dural sac ends at S2/S3. However, the anatomy of the sacral hiatus is quite variable.

Technique
The patient assumes a semi-prone or prone position and the sacral hiatus is located between the sacral promontories. A weal is raised and the needle (large- or fine-bore) is inserted perpendicularly through the sacrococcygeal membrane and advanced until contact is made with the posterior aspect of the sacral body. Withdraw slightly and deflect the hub of the needle into the natal cleft, advance 1–2 cm and test for position (aspiration and loss of resistance to air). Local anaesthetic is injected (10–20 ml).

Hazards additional to those of lumbar epidural
- Possible increased risk of infection
- Danger of injury to fetus if carried out during the second stage of labour

PUDENDAL (FIG. 4.7)

S2, S3 and S4 join to form the pudendal nerve 0.5–1.0 cm proximal to the ischial spine. It then passes posteriorly to the spines between the sacrospinous and sacrotuberous ligaments. That is,

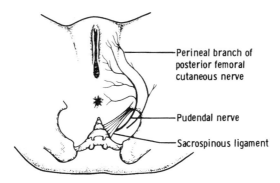

Perineal branch of posterior femoral cutaneous nerve

Pudendal nerve

Sacrospinous ligament

Fig 4.7   The courses of the pudendal and perineal nerves

it passes from the greater sciatic notch to the lesser sciatic notch. Of inferior haemorrhoidal nerves, 50% arise directly from the sacral plexus; they perforate the sacrospinous ligament and lie close to the tip of the ischial spine.

Transperineal approach:
With the patient in the lithotomy position a skin weal is made 2/3 of the way from the anus to the ischial tuberosity. The ischial spine is palpated from within the vagina and a 10 cm needle is directed through the weal to a point just inferior to the spine. After an aspiration test, 10 ml of local anaesthetic is injected.

Transvaginal approach:
A sheathed needle is held between the first and second fingers and advanced into the vagina until the ischial spine and sacrospinous ligament are palpated by the second finger. The needle is inserted 1 cm at a point 1 cm medial to the spine and 1 cm below the lower edge of the ligament. Then 10 ml of local anaesthetic is injected.

The perineal branch of the posterior femoral cutaneous nerve is blocked at the latero-posterior aspect of the ischial tuberosity (5 ml) and the episiotomy line should be infiltrated (5 ml).

This is a poor method for producing pain-relief in labour. High concentrations of local anaesthetic cause relaxation of the pelvic diaphragm which reduces the mother's ability to assist expulsion of the fetus.

PARACERVICAL

A sheathed needle is inserted into the right and left fornices of the vagina, the needle is then advanced 1–2 cm and 5–10 ml of local anaesthetic is injected after a negative aspiration test.

Sensory nerves are blocked as they pass through the broad ligaments; however, the number that pass by that route is variable. Uterine efficiency is not diminished.

Fetal bradycardia, tachycardia and acidosis have all been reported and may be due to either direct toxic effects or to a reduction in placental perfusion consequent upon depression of the maternal circulation.

A success rate of between 55% and 85%, high concentrations of local anaesthetic entering the fetal circulation and an inability to initiate the block in the 2nd stage of labour make this a technique of dubious value.

NERVE BLOCKS FOR SURGERY OF THE LIMBS

Arm: Brachial plexus block
        Circumferential block
        Intravenous block

Leg: Lumbar plexus block
        Sacral plexus block
        Circumferential block
        Intravenous block

ARM

Brachial plexus block

1. Interscalene technique
Position the patient supine with the head turned to the contra-lateral side. A finger is placed between the sternocleidomastoid muscle, at the level of the 6th cervical vertebra, resting on the anterior scalene muscle. A needle is inserted into this groove, perpendicular to the skin, and advanced until the paraesthesia are elicited. Aspirate, and inject the local anaesthetic if satisfactory. Pneumothorax is not a complication.

2. Supraclavicular technique
There are many techniques, but care must be taken to avoid pneumothorax. The 'parascalene technique' (Vongvises and Panijnyanond) has been described recently.
     The patient lies supine, with the head turned to face away from the side to be treated, and with the arms by the side. A finger is placed immediately lateral to the sternocleidomastoid, immediately above the clavicle. It will lie on scalenus anterior which is moved laterally. A needle is inserted 3 cm in an antero-posterior direction, 2 cm above the clavicle and immediately lateral to the anterior scalene muscle. When paraesthesia is elicited, aspirate; if satisfactory, inject local anaesthetic. If the needle strikes bone (the first rib) without paraesthesia, inject local anaesthetic in a fan-like manner.

3. Infraclavicular technique
An advantage with this technique is that the intercosto-brachial nerve (T2) is blocked (Fig. 4.8).
     The patient lies supine with the head turned face-away from the side that is to be blocked. A needle is inserted 2.5 cm below the midpoint of the clavicle and advanced laterally towards the brachial artery. Use a peripheral nerve stimulator to confirm the correct position.

4. Axillary technique
Pneumothorax is not a complication of this technique; however, there is usually anaesthesia of only the lower arm.
Musculocutaneous nerve blockade may be achieved by using larger volumes of local anaesthetic.
     The supine patient abducts the arm to a right angle and the humerus is externally rotated by placing the hand behind the head.

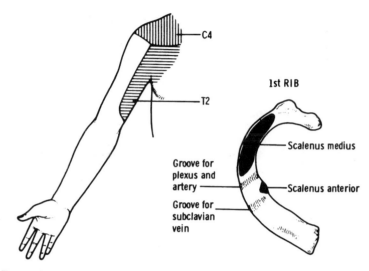

Fig 4.8   Important anatomical structures for brachial plexus block

A needle is inserted above the artery, high up in the axilla at the level of the lower margin of pectoralis major. A change in resistance to pressure identifies the passage through the fascial sheath; paraesthesia may be elicited. The brachial artery is compressed below the site of the injection to occlude the neuro-vascular sheath distally, and local anaesthetic is injected. After withdrawing the needle the arm is adducted, maintaining pressure over the brachial artery distal. Local anaesthetic is now injected. Adduction of the arm is said to release the occlusion of the neurovascular sheath proximal to the site of injection, by the head of humerus, allowing proximal spread of the local anaesthetic, which makes a block of the musculocutaneous nerve more likely.

Circumferential blocks
Circumferential blocks may be achieved at the elbow and wrist by subcutaneous and intradermal infiltration. Depots of local anaesthetic should be injected in the appropriate positions to block the median, radial and ulnar nerves.

Intravenous blocks (Bier)

Technique:
Insert a cannula into a vein on the dorsum of the hand (a needle is more likely to pierce the vein during the subsequent manoeuvres). A second intravenous cannula must be inserted into a vein on the opposite side. A double-cuff tourniquet is positioned on the upper

arm. The arm may now be elevated, a roller or an Esmarch bandage applied. If the latter, premedication or some form of analgesia may be necessary. Inflate the proximal cuff on the tourniquet above systolic blood pressure. The local anaesthetic solution without adrenaline is injected—up to a volume of 40 ml of 0.5% lignocaine, or prilocaine for a fit 70 kg man (for an arm)—and the solution is massaged into peripheral areas, as the finger tips often retain sensation.

The distal cuff is inflated, and the proximal cuff deflated, strictly in that order. This protects the patient against leak of the local anaesthetic into the systemic circulation, and reduces the pain associated with the tourniquet as the pressure is now applied over an area that has been subject to the action of the local anaesthetic. If a bloodless field is required the tourniquet remains applied, otherwise it may be deflated gradually after the drug is fixed in the tissues (at least 20 minutes). Analgesia does not persist for very long once the cuff is deflated. The local anaesthetic may seep past the tourniquet through venous channels in bone. (Hence do not use Bupivacaine.)

Contraindications
• Poor patient cooperation
• Infection in limb
• Surgical duration greater than one hour
• Allergy to local anaesthesia
• Single tourniquet
• Sickle cell trait or disease
• Raynaud's disease

LEG

Lumbar plexus
• Iliohypogastric
• Ilioinguinal
• Genitofemoral
• Lateral cutaneous nerve of thigh
• Obturator
• Femoral

These nerves pass between the quadratus lumborum and psoas muscles, and an extension of their investing fascial sheath may be used to direct the local anaesthetic agent to block the whole plexus: the 'inguinal paravascular technique' (Winnie).

A needle is inserted lateral to the femoral artery and when paraesthesia is elicited in the distribution of the femoral nerve the local anaesthetic is injected. The drug will pass up the fascial cleft and block the lumbar plexus. (Alternative techniques involve multiple blocks.)

Sacral plexus
- Sciatic nerve (Fig. 4.9)
- Posterior cutaneous nerve
- Pudendal nerve

The sciatic and posterior cutaneous nerve of thigh leave the pelvis together and a block of the sciatic nerve results in a block of the latter also. Only the pudendal then remains to be blocked.

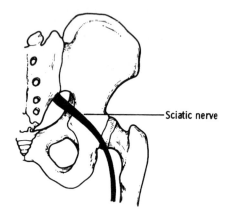

Sciatic nerve

Fig 4.9   The course of the sciatic nerve in the region of the hip

Posterior (Labat) technique
A needle is inserted 5–7.5 cm deep at a point 3 cm below the midpoint of a line joining the posterior iliac spine and the greater trochanter. Then 10–15 ml of local anaesthetic is injected.

Anterior (Beck) technique
A line is drawn from the greater trochanter parallel with the inguinal ligament. Another line is drawn perpendicular to the first from a point two thirds of the way along the inguinal ligament from the anterior superior iliac spine. At this point a needle is inserted to pass on the medial side of the femur, and 20–30 ml of local anaesthetic is injected.

Lateral (Ichiyanagy) technique
The patient lies supine with a pillow below the knee. A line is drawn along the shaft of the femur to pass through the posterior border of the greater trochanter. Then, 2 cm beyond the trochanter a needle is inserted 10–15 cm in the horizontal plane. Paraesthesia should be elicited.

Note: Both the lumbar and sacral plexus may be blocked by a lumbar paravertebral approach: see p. 130.

Circumferential blocks
A circumferential block may be achieved at the ankle. Infiltrate both subcutaneous and intradermal tissues. Depots of local anaesthetic are injected to block the sural, saphenous and medial popliteal nerves at the ankle. The lateral popliteal nerve is blocked near the neck of the fibula.

Intravenous block (Bier)
The technique in the leg is similar to that performed in the arm. A large volume, up to 80 ml, of local anaesthetic solution should be used to ensure adequate dispersal of the agent.

CHRONIC PAIN
Pain, which has been inadequately defined as the sensation normally experienced in response to a noxious stimulus, is the symptom that most commonly causes the patient to seek medical advice. Pain of a chronic and excruciating nature is both demoralising and incapacitating. The management of chronic pain requires a flexible, multidisciplinary approach and skills in psychotherapy, neurology and local analgesia techniques may be required.

Pain is a subjective experience and a complaint of pain should never be attributed to imagination or 'nerves'. Exhaustive investigation may eventually uncover an organic cause for the pain.

There are four types of chronic pain:
1. Inflammatory pain
2. Neural damage pain
3. Sympathetic pain
4. Psychological pain

Treatment
1. Analgesics
2. Adjuvants
3. Amitriptyline
4. NSAIDs
5. Local anaesthetics
6. Steroids
7. Chemical neurolysis
8. Transcutaneous electrical nerve stimulation (TENS)
9. Percutaneous electrical neurolysis
10. Acupuncture
11. Hypnosis

1. Analgesics should be chosen so that pain relief is with minimal adverse effects. Some adverse effects may be acceptable for patients with terminal conditions though not for the patient with benign lesions.

BENIGN CHRONIC PAIN	PAINFUL TERMINAL CONDITIONS
Analgesia without sedation	Analgesia ± sedation and euphoria
Analgesia without addiction	Addiction not an absolute contraindication
Oral preparation	
Avoid emesis and constipation	Oral, i.m. or i.v.
	Control emesis and constipation, if necessary, with adjuvant agents

Analgesics should be taken at regular intervals so that the pain does not return. Taking painkillers 'as required' is usually less effective.

2. Antidepressants and/or tranquillisers are used as adjuvants. Chlorpromazine has a potentiating effect on analgesics. It is also antiemetic and sedative. Antidepressant therapy almost always decreases the analgesic requirements for those with terminal therapy.
3. Amitriptyline is effective for post-herpetic neuralgia and diabetic neuropathy. Anticonvulsants (sodium valproate) are effective for trigeminal neuralgia. Other useful drugs include clonidine, carbamazine and flecainide. Phantom limb pain may be treated with clonazepam or anticonvulsants.
4. Oral NSAIDs progress to combinations of NSAID and opioid and combinations which are additive. Dose of opioid may be increased if pain control inadequate. Watch for constipation, nausea and vomiting and drowsiness.
5. The injection of local anaesthetics into painful areas, or to block the somatic nerves serving those areas, may have a duration of effect far greater than that due to their pharmacokinetic properties. One hypothesis is that a vicious circle of pain–muscle spasm–pain may be broken by the single injection and thus produce permanent pain relief.
6. Steroid preparations may be mixed with local anaesthetic to infiltrate painful sites. Their anti-flammatory property abates the cause of the pain. Epidural local anaesthesia/steroid mixtures have been used for pain associated with vertebral disc lesions.
7. Chemical neurolysis produces a permanent or prolonged block of pain pathways. The two commonly used agents are 5% phenol in glycerine and 50% alcohol in water. 5% phenol destroys C fibres and preserves the larger A fibres. Alcohol is painful on injection and can cause persistent pain by causing a neuritis. It is used for sympathetic blocks and for pituitary ablation.
   a. Somatic nerve blockade
      When using neurolytic agents on somatic nerves the motor function of the nerve to be blocked must be considered; a block of C2 and T2 to T12, has little serious outcome. The pain fibres (C) which are smaller in diameter and unmyelinated are more susceptible to neurolysis than the motor (A) fibres.

b. Sympathetic blockade
Sympathetic tone may be reduced by suitable blockade.
This also reduces pain due to excessive sympathetic tone,
and also blocks C fibres, which travel with the sympathetic
nerves.
Conditions relieved by appropriate sympathetic blockade:
- Sympathetic reflex dystrophy
  — Causalgia—pain, hyperaesthesia, vasospasm
  — Thalamic pain
  — Phantom limb pain
  — Shoulder–hand syndrome
  — Sudek's atrophy
  — Post-frostbite syndrome
  — Post-traumatic pain syndrome
  — Post-traumatic oedema
- Vascular disorders
  — Raynaud's disease
  — Thrombophlebitis
  — Emboli
  — Vasospasm
  — Intermittent claudication
- Pain associated with carcinoma of the stomach, lung, gall bladder,
  spleen or pancreas (coeliac plexus block)
  c. Subarachnoid blocks
  Careful subarachnoid injection of neurolytic agents can
  produce an effect confined to the dorsal nerve root and thus
  avoid motor effects; the patient must be kept tilted to the
  appropriate side for 1 hour after the injection. When C3–T1
  and L1–S3 are involved possible damage to nerve function
  and sphincter control must be weighed against the
  advantages to be gained. 2% chlorocresol or 5% phenol, in
  glycerine, is used for subarachnoid injection; there are
  hyperbaric solutions.
  d. Pituitary ablation
  Pituitary ablation has been found to relieve pain completely
  in 40% of patients with disseminated metastatic pain. 1 ml
  of absolute alcohol is injected through a transphenoidal
  needle into the pituitary gland.
8. Transcutaneous electrical nerve stimulation (TENS) produces
   pain relief by applying the 'gate' theory of pain to the clinical
   situation. The large-fibre activity is increased and by balancing
   large- and small-fibre activity the 'gate' closes. Electrical
   current is applied through pads strapped to the skin and is
   effective for a variety of chronic pain situations.
9. Percutaneous electrical neurolysis/cordotomy
   Radio-frequency-generated heat lesions in the antero-lateral
   spinothalamic tract can produce pain relief on the contralateral
   side below the level of the lesion. A needle is passed between
   the first and second cervical vertebrae, and advanced to

penetrate the anterior lateral aspect of the cord (Fig. 4.10). Small stimulating electric currents aid the positioning of the needle before the heat lesion is produced. Cryo-probes are used to create lesions; the very low temperatures (–60°C) are achieved by the sudden expansion of gas under pressure— adiabatic expansion.

10. Acupuncture (a Chinese method for pain relief) is achieved by 'twiddling' of, or electrical stimulation of, fine needles positioned in the skin at specific locations. It is thought that the needles cause the release of endogenous opiate-like substances, found useful for the management of persistent pain. Not everyone responds to acupuncture.

11. Hypnosis in the responsive patient may be an alternative method of pain relief. However, the analgesic effect of hypnosis diminishes when used over a prolonged period. Patients can be trained to initiate self-hypnosis.

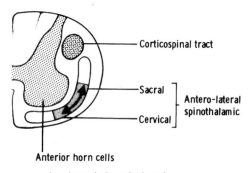

Fig 4.10   Transverse section through the spinal cord

POSTOPERATIVE ANALGESIA

The advantages and disadvantages of the various methods are given in Table 4.1.

Methods in common use
- Oral analgesics
- Intramuscular analgesic injection
- Local anaesthetic (L.A.) and regional (epidural) opiate techniques

Other methods
- Cryo-analgesia
- Intravenous analgesia
- Nitrous oxide inhalation
- Transcutaneous electrical nerve stimulation
- Acupuncture
- Hypnosis

Table 4.1

Method	Advantages	Disadvantages
i.m.	Convenience. Acute overdose unlikely.	Fluctuating levels of analgesia, repeated injection and given at the nurse's discretion.
Oral	No injections, facilitates discharge home (day cases)	Absorption variable. Not suitable following gastrointestinal surgery. Fluctuating analgesia.
L.A. epidural opiates	Almost continuous analgesia possible. Profound analgesia permits coughing.	All complications associated with L.A. Medically qualified practitioner required for 'top-ups'. Possible hypotension and loss of motor power with L.A.; skin itching and late respiratory depression if opiates used.
Cryo-analgesia	Reduces use of drugs.	Restricted to post-thoracotomy pain. However, thoracotomy pain is of diverse origins, and pain relief may be incomplete.
i.v.	Titration of dose. Continuous analgesia. Patient-controlled demand systems are available.	Acute overdose possible. Expensive equipment is required per patient. Care and attention of intravenous line necessary.
Nitrous oxide	Continuous analgesia. Pulmonary performance improved. Use for dressing changes.	Pollution. Danger of bone marrow depression after 48 hours' continuous use.
TENS	Avoids depressant drugs.	Controlled trials impossible but its efficacy is not high.
Acupuncture/ Hypnosis	Avoids depressant drugs.	Time-consuming. Low efficacy.

Pain is a subjective experience and is influenced by many factors that are not easily measured.

GENERAL COMMENTS

1. Morphine is the standard analgesic with which others are compared.
2. Approximately one-third of patients obtain relief from a placebo, though usually for less time than from an active drug.
3. Increasing the dose of an agent may not necessarily increase analgesia, but the side-effects are increased.
4. It is better to repeat analgesics before pain returns.

5. General discomfort accentuates pain.
6. Good general analgesia may not protect the patient from pain associated with coughing or physiotherapy.
7. Some patients experience greater pain than others.
   Neurotics > extroverts
   Central operations > peripheral operations
8. The use of local anaesthetic techniques to provide postoperative analgesia may not markedly enhance respiratory function, although coughing and physiotherapy are less painful (intercostal block may be superior to epidural block as hypotension and urinary retention may follow an epidural—however, pneumothorax is a risk).
9. Logistics usually determines the method of pain control used.

ANATOMY OF SPINE, EPIDURAL SPACE AND SPINAL CORD

33 vertebrae—7 cervical, 12 thoracic, 5 lumbar, 5 sacral, 4 coccygeal

Vertebra
• Body
• Vertebral arch
• Pedicles—grooved to form the intervertebral foraminae
• Laminae
• Transverse and spinal processes
• Articular facets

• Cervical — 1,2,7, atypical–vertebral foramen–artery, vein and sympathetic nerves
• Thoracic — 1,2,3,4, spines horizontal to oblique
  5,6,7,8, spines almost vertical
  9,10,11,12, oblique to horizontal
  } Articular facets for ribs
• Lumbar — 1,2,3,4,5, No rib facets, no vertebral foramen. Body taller in front than behind; heavy spines horizontal.

Ligaments
• Anterior longitudinal ligament—axis to sacrum
• Posterior longitudinal ligament—axis to sacrum
• Ligament flavum—yellow elastic fibres from the articular facets to spinal processes and from the anterior inferior aspect of lamina above to the posterior superior aspect of lamina below
• There is a midline cleft between ligamenta flava
• Inter-spinous ligament—connects the spinous processes from root to tip, fusing with the ligamenta flava
• Supra-spinous ligament—a continuation of the ligamentum nuchae C7 to sacrum

Intervertebral discs
These comprise a quarter of the spine length, act as shock absorbers and are composed of the annulus fibrosus and nucleus pulposus.

Spinal cord and coverings
- Medulla oblongata to L1/2 (neonate L3)
- Cauda equina
- Filum terminale interna—thread-like extension or cord, ends with dura and arachnoid at S2—continues as filum terminale externa which blends with the periosteum of the coccyx.
- Dura mater, arachnoid, pia mater
  The dura mater is composed of periosteal and investing layers, the latter covers the spinal cord and the former lines the spinal canal. The potential space between the two layers is called the extradual, epidural, or, perhaps more correctly, the interdural space.

EPIDURAL SPACE

Foramen magnum is the upper limit of the space and the sacral hiatus is the lower. Dural cuffs cover the spinal nerves which pass through the intervertebral foraminae into the paravertebral space. The epidural space is greatest at mid-thoracic level (6 mm).

There are both anterior and posterior venous plexuses and these connect with the intervertebral veins; together they form venous rings at the level of each vertebra.

Branches from the vertebral, ascending cervical, deep cervical, intercostal, lumbar and ilio-lumbar arteries also enter the intervertebral foramina and anastomose in the lateral aspects of the epidural space. The epidural space also contains fat tissue.

PHYSIOLOGICAL EFFECTS OF SPINAL/EPIDURAL BLOCKADE

NERVE CONDUCTION

Pre-ganglionic sympathetic fibres are blocked first. In increasing order of fibre diameter the sensory modalities are blocked; temperature, pain, touch, pressure and then the motor fibres are blocked followed by the proprioceptor pathways.

VASCULAR

- Loss of sympathetic tone
- Venous pooling due to lack of skeletal muscle tone
- Fall in central venous pressure, cardiac output falls
- Blood pressure falls

RESPIRATORY

- Spinal—cephalic spread of local anaesthetic may block intercostal nerves, or, if higher, the phrenic nerves causing apnoea
- Epidural—respiratory paralysis very unlikely but pain relief more likely to improve ventilation

GASTROINTESTINAL TRACT

The bowel contracts and the sphincters relax. Nausea and retching may still occur.

5. Intensive care

The intensive care (or therapy) unit (ITU) is costly on medical and nursing staff and also an financial resources. Attempts have therefore been made over the years to better define the admission criteria and progress using scoring systems. Of the many available, the best known, and probably the most reliable, is the APACHE system, currently in its third generation. Most body organ systems can be supported in the ITU, although the more that fail the worse is the prognosis. Failure of four systems or more has a mortality of almost 100%.

The ITU is a complex, noisy and frightening environment into which to bring a patient. It is common therefore to sedate almost all patients, at least for the first few hours or days. There are no hard and fast rules for sedation except that all patients who receive a muscle relaxant must be adequately sedated. There is no way of monitoring sedation except for subjective scoring systems, e.g. the Ramsey scale. Every patient has different needs and so must be managed individually.

Most sedation regimes centre around the continuous infusion of an opioid (e.g. morphine, fentanyl or alfentanil) together with either midazolam or propofol. Ketamine and isoflurane have also been used for specific situations. Large textbooks exist which are devoted to management of the critically ill patient. This short chapter therefore only covers the more common situations in brief and uses them to illustrate basic principles of intensive care.

MANAGEMENT OF HEAD INJURIES

Mild head injuries without loss of consciousness or with only a short temporary loss of consciousness and no structural damage to the brain are usually dealt with by the accident and emergency physicians with input from the neurosurgeons and possible overnight admission if there are any complicating issues, e.g. pre-existing significant medical history or there is no responsible adult to escort the patient home. This section concerns the more severe head injury characterised by a prolonged loss of consciousness, or a continuing impaired level of consciousness, and is often associated with structural damage to the brain. Management can be divided into four broad areas: assessment, general supportive measures, specific therapy, monitoring. Remember that resuscitation is the first priority and should take place before and continue during the assessment period.

ASSESSMENT

1. Conscious level
Conscious level is usually assessed by scoring responses of the

patient to verbal commands and painful stimuli. The universal
scoring system is the Glasgow coma scale (Table 5.1) which can be
repeated at intervals to give a measure of any changing level of
consciousness.

Table 5.1   The Glasgow coma scale

Test	Reaction	Score
Eye opening	Spontaneously	4
	To command	3
	To pain	2
	None	1
Best verbal response	Orientated	5
	Confused	4
	Inappropriate	3
	Incomprehensible	2
	None	1
Best motor response	Obeys commands	6
	Localises to pain	5
	Flexes to pain	4
	Abnormal flexion or rigidity to pain	3
	Extends to pain	2
	None	1

Note
Maximum score is 15; minimum score is 3.

2. Pupil size and reactivity
Sluggish or absent pupillary light reflexes may indicate a significant
brain injury or possibly ingestion of a poison. Differences in
reactivity between the two sides may point to a localising injury.
Regular charting of pupillary reflexes (every 15 min if necessary)
may give an early indication of a progressing lesion.

3. Spontaneous muscle movements and convulsions
The character and location should be regularly charted because
they may give a clue as to the nature and progression of the injury.
Muscle tone, reflexes, abnormal posturing and decerebrate rigidity
should also be recorded.

4. Temperature
The patient's temperature—preferably core—should be measured
at intervals. Impairment of thermal homeostasis may be associated
with a poor prognosis. Hypertension may indicate the ingestion of
a stimulant drug.

5. Cardiovascular and respiratory status
Hypoxia and hypotension increase the morbidity following a head
injury. Good oxygenation (if necessary intubate and ventilate) and

maintenance of cerebral perfusion pressure (fluid, inotropes, etc. as required) are essential.

6. *Exclude other causes of coma, e.g. drugs, alcohol, diabetes, CVA*
A thorough examination must be undertaken to determine whether any other injuries are present. The presence of thoracic or upper abdominal trauma markedly increases the morbidity and mortality. Head injury is often associated with injuries to the cervical spine.

GENERAL SUPPORTIVE MEASURES

1. Maintenance of the airway. Position the patient approximately and, if necessary, insert an oropharyngeal airway. If there is any doubt, insert an oral endotracheal tube to both protect and maintain the airway. Avoid coughing and straining. Beware of possible cervical spine injury.
2. Maintenance of ventilation. The F_1O_2 may require increasing if the P_aO_2 falls. Patients with head injuries are prone to pulmonary oedema. Measure the blood gases regularly.
3. The blood pressure must be maintained (and therefore the cerebral perfusion pressure) but overhydration should be avoided. Shock implies trauma and bleeding elsewhere.
4. Control of restlessness and convulsions. Propofol administered by infusion is useful as return to the patient's unsedated state occurs rapidly once the infusion is stopped, allowing reassessment within a short time. Muscle relaxants may be required but convulsions should be controlled first.
5. Feeding should be instituted after 24 hours. Avoid overhydration as the blood/brain barrier is damaged and cerebral oedema occurs easily.

SPECIFIC THERAPY

1. Control of intracranial pressure
   a. Reduction of fluid intake will tend to decrease intracranial pressure, but beware of hypovolaemia.
   b. Osmotic dehydrating agents may be used. They are not definitive treatment as there may be a rebound phenomenon, which occurs after a variable period of time, depending on the agent used. This results in a subsequent increase in intracranial pressure. Leakage of the agent into a haematoma may increase its size.
   c. Steroids are no longer used. Diabetes insipidus will require treatment with DDAVP.
   d. Intermittent positive pressure ventilation is used to lower the P_aCO_2 (aim for 4–4.3 kPa) and this in turn reduces the intracranial pressure. A P_aCO_2 below 3.5 kPa may increase cerebral hypoxia secondary to cerebral vasoconstriction. Damaged brain tissue does not respond to changes in carbon

dioxide tension and thus will tend to remain well perfused ('luxury' perfusion) when the P_aCO_2 is low. If the P_aCO_2 is high, the reverse occurs and the normal brain 'steals' blood flow from the damaged area which cannot respond by vasodilation.

    e. Surgical relief of the raised intracranial pressure by burr hole or craniotomy. A shunt may be required.

2. To limit or reduce further damage

    a. Hypothermia may be of use if the patient is hyperthermic but the overall results are not encouraging: the number of survivors increases, though frequently in a vegetative state.

    b. It has been shown in animals that large doses of barbiturates may protect the brain against hypoxic damage, reduce ICP and control convulsions. Care must be taken not to depress the cardiovascular system and thus reduce cerebral perfusion pressure.

    c. Control convulsions. Phenytoin is the drug of choice.

MONITORING

1. Routine monitoring of cardiovascular and respiratory function
2. Temperature
3. Fluid balance
4. Neurosurgical assessment charts. See Table 5.1. Repeat as often as necessary—every 15 minutes if needed.
5. Intracranial pressure. The intracranial pressure may be measured directly by placing a cannula in the extradural, subdural or intraventricular space. Subdural and intraventricular techniques share the possibility of introducing infection. Extradural techniques, while losing a degree of sensitivity, reduce the incidence of infection. A number of newer systems have been developed which use fibreoptic technology. Intracranial pressure monitoring is used more often in current practice due to the greater accuracy of modern equipment and also because of evidence which suggests that tighter control of intracranial pressure and cerebral perfusion pressure reduces morbidity.

CIRCULATORY FAILURE AND CARDIOVASCULAR SUPPORT

DIAGNOSIS

- Hypotension, tachycardia
- Confusion or unconsciousness
- Oliguria or anuria
- Cold periphery with raised core temperature

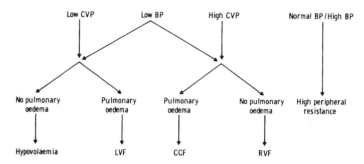

Fig 5.1 Differentiation of the causes of poor perfusion

CAUSES

- Relative or absolute hypovolaemia
- Pump failure—right-sided, left-sided, or both.
  These functional causes may result from many processes, each requiring specific treatment. Common causes include:
- Trauma—severe haemorrhage, external or internal
- Burns—loss of plasma
- Bacteraemia—Gram negative endotoxaemia (periphery may be warm)
- Heart failure—myocardial infarction, pulmonary embolism, cardiac tamponade
- Neurogenic—sympathetic inhibition, intracranial haemorrhage
- Miscellaneous—electrolyte and fluid loss (vomiting and diarrhoea)

TREATMENT

This is designed, with regard to aetiology:
1. Increase cardiac output by increasing circulating volume or by using inotropic agents
2. Raise P_aO_2 by increasing F_1O_2 (may require IPPV)
3. Eliminate infection
4. Sustain renal function

In the majority of situations the cause can be determined by central venous pressure (CVP) measurement and measurement of systolic blood pressure (SBP), e.g. low CVP and low SBP suggests relative or absolute hypovolaemia; high CVP and low SBP suggests pump failure. (Fig. 5.1)

ASSESSMENT AND TREATMENT OF HYPOVOLAEMIA

A dynamic assessment of central venous pressure should be made. A volume of fluid (e.g. 100–200 ml of saline) is infused

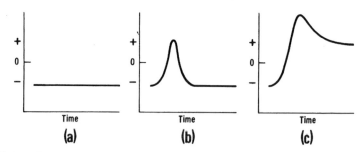

Fig 5.2 Dynamic testing of the central venous pressure

quickly and the response of the CVP monitored. No change in CVP suggests a marked hypovolaemia (Fig. 5.2a). A transient rise in CVP which falls quickly indicates moderate hypovolaemia (Fig. 5.2b) and a large rise in CVP with a slow fall indicates an adequately filled cardiovascular system (Fig. 5.2c). Several litres of fluid may be required to replace volume deficit.

After the first testing of the circulatory status with saline, a colloid of longer intravascular persistence is indicated. If the cause of the perfusion failure is hypovolaemia, then heart rate, blood pressure, urine output and temperature will all respond quickly to adequate fluid replacement. The adequacy of fluid replacement may be confirmed by identifying the response to further aliquots of fluid.

BLOOD VOLUME EXPANSION

Transfusion of compatible blood is used for volume espansion, if blood loss is the problem. Circulatory volume may be increased temporarily by the use of crystalloids in a dire emergency associated with haemorrhage. Circulating volume may be increased for a longer period by the use of colloid solutions which include;

1. Human albumin solution (4.5%—there is no hepatitis risk and it is ABO-compatible but expensive)
2. Concentrated albumin (25% albumin in water; oncotic pressure = oncotic pressure of plasma × 5)
3. Degraded starch solutions (hetastarch or pentastarch)
4. Gelatin solutions (anaphylactoid reactions are possible)

ASSESSMENT AND MANAGEMENT OF PUMP FAILURE

The outflow of blood from the right side must equal the outflow from the left side of the heart. Different end diastolic pressures (roughly equivalent to CVP and left atrial pressure respectively) are required to produce the same stroke volume in the two ventricles (Fig. 5.3). In the normal heart a CVP of 10 will produce an equivalent right ventricular stroke volume to that produced by 5 cmH$_2$O in the left ventricle.

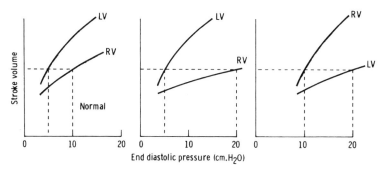

Fig 5.3 End diastolic pressure/stroke volume relations in the heart

A failing right ventricle requires a greater CVP to produce the same stroke volume. In left ventricular failure a higher filling pressure is also required. If the driving pressure required to produce an adequate stroke volume/cardiac output is greater than 20 cmH$_2$O, however, then the oncotic pressure of the pulmonary circulation is exceeded and pulmonary oedema occurs. Pump failure can therefore usually be differentiated by CVP and BP determination and the absence or presence of pulmonary oedema.

Catheterisation of the pulmonary artery, using a flow-directed catheter, allows measurement of the pulmonary artery pressure, cardiac output and pulmonary capillary wedge pressure (PCWP). The PCWP reflects the filling pressures of the left atrium and therefore the left ventricular end diastolic pressure (LVEDP) can be estimated. In the presence of severe left sided heart failure the PCWP may exceed 20 mmHg but be less than the LVEDP. Pulmonary artery catheterisation also permits the arteriovenous oxygen difference to be determined.

The management of pump failure has several important facets:
1. Control of contractility and heart rate
2. Maintenance of oxygen supply/oxygen demand ratio > 1
3. Control of preload and afterload

INOTROPIC AGENTS

Cardiac glycosides—e.g. digoxin, digitoxin, ovabaine
There are a large number of active glycosides which increase the stroke volume, diastolic volume and a stroke work for a given

filling pressure. Cardiac slowing results from central vagal stimulation with peripheral potentiation of vagal effect. In addition there is reduced atrio-ventricular conduction.

Inhibition of membrane-bound ATP occurs, thus inhibiting the sodium pump and allowing sodium to flow into the cell and potassium to flow out. The resulting increase in intracellular sodium may facilitate the entry of calcium with a resultant inotropic effect. The fall in intracellular potassium slows atrio-ventricular conduction and sensitises the sinus node to vagal stimulation.

Dopamine

Dopamine is the penultimate step in the biosynthesis of noradrenaline. Dopamine is a neurotransmitter in its own right and is released by dopaminergic fibres. It stimulates alpha and beta adrenoceptors and dopamine receptors. Dopamine infused at 2–5 mg.kg^{-1}min^{-1} produces vasodilation of the mesenteric and renal vessels. At 5–10 mg.kg^{-1}.min^{-1} it has an inotropic effect and increases the heart rate. A dose of > 15 mg.kg^{-1}min^{-1} produces vasoconstriction. It has been replaced by other vasoactive amines and is now not often used.

Dobutamine

A beta-adrenergic inotrope, dobutamine may produce a tachycardia in high doses. It is more selective than dopamine and better at increasing myocardial contractility and thus cardiac output. It is the first-line inotrope of choice in most ITUs.

Dopexamine

This synthetic catecholamine has activity at adrenergic beta-2 and dopamine-1 receptors. It also inhibits the noradrenaline reuptake-1 mechanism. It has been described as an inodilator because it produces both an inotropic effect and a vasodilator effect. The vasodilator effect is principally seen in the mesenteric and renal vascular beds and dopexamine has superseded dopamine in many ITUs. It occasionally produces a troublesome and persistent tachycardia which limits the dose.

PHOSPHODIESTERASE INHIBITORS

These drugs have an effect which is not mediated via the beta receptors and should, theoretically, be unaffected by down-regulation of receptors. They are inotopes but also augment relaxation and filling of the left ventricle. It was originally believed that these agents improved myocardial performance without affecting myocardial oxygen consumption. Some doubt has been expressed with respect to this claim, however.

The different drugs available within this family (e.g. enoximone, milrionone, amrinone) do not have exactly identical actions, probably due to both pharmacokinetic differences and to the different isoenzymes of phosphodiesterase which exist. They all possess both inotropic and vasodilator actions, the predominant effect of which may be difficult to predict. A troublesome tachycardia may develop.

Vasodilators (arterial and venous)
Vasodilator drugs may significantly increase vascular capacity and thereby endanger cerebral and coronary artery blood flow. If, in spite of a normal or raised blood pressure, tissue perfusion is poor the use of a vasodilating agent may improve peripheral perfusion by reducing vasoconstriction. Sodium nitroprusside, which primarily reduces afterload, is useful in the presence of a raised blood pressure and a low or normal PCWP. Glyceryl trinitrate, primarily a venodilator, reduces preload and is useful in patients with myocardial ischaemia (the end diastolic pressure is lower and therefore so is the ventricular wall tension—myocardial perfusion is thus enhanced).

The precapillary sphincter constricts in response to catecholamines and the postcapillary sphincter in response to hypoxaemia and an associated fall in pH. Constriction of the precapillary sphincter will ultimately produce contraction of the postcapillary sphincter because of reduced oxygen delivery. Constricted peripheral arterioles, with pre- and postcapillary sphincter constriction, reduce tissue perfusion and thereby worsen tissue hypoxia. Relaxation of the arterioles using vasoactive drugs, accompanied by efficient oxygenation, will cause relaxation of the venous sphincters. If this does not occur pooling of blood within the capillary network will occur.

The reduction in peripheral resistance resulting from alpha blockade may improve left ventricular function by decreasing the afterload; however, a fall in blood pressure—particularly diastolic—also reduces oxygen delivery to the myocardium.

RESPIRATORY FAILURE AND VENTILATORY SUPPORT

Respiratory failure is defined as the inability to maintain normal (for the patient) ventilatory function or acceptable blood gases. There are many aetiological factors, the commonest of which are given in Table 5.2. Hypoxia may occur, with or without hypercarbia, and may be related to respiratory disease, cardiac disease, or diseases in another system. Upper or lower airway disease (e.g. tracheal obstruction, exess secretions and ventilation perfusion disturbances (e.g. atelectasis, pulmonary emboli) may result in respiratory failure.

Table 5.2   Causes of respiratory failure

System	Causes
Acute lung disease	Bronchopneumonia
	Lobar pneumonia
	Acute or chronic bronchitis
	Emphysema
	Industrial lung disease
	Asthma
	Kyphoscoliosis
	Fractured ribs
	Pneumothorax, haemothorax
	Pleural effusion
Nerves and muscles	Guillain-Barré syndrome
	Myasthenia gravis
	Tetanus
	Neuromuscular blocking agents
	Demyelinating diseases
Central nervous system	Poisoning, drugs
	Hypoxaemia
	Infection
	Trauma
	Tumour
	Poliomyelitis
	Raised ICP

Oxygen therapy

Hypoxia requires oxygen administration and is usually without hazard. However, the patient whose ventilatory drive depends largely on a low oxygen tension and the patient who requires prolonged administration of a very high concentration of oxygen may be at risk.

The classic 'blue bloater' is not common but oxygen therapy may reduce hypoxic respiratory drive and thus lead, if undiagnosed, to hypercarbia. The inspired oxygen concentration must be titrated, generally between 25% and 30% which increases O_2 saturation but with only a minimal increase in P_aO_2. Oxygen toxicity from damage to the alveolar cells may result from breathing high partial pressure of oxygen. The administration of high oxygen concentrations to premature babies may lead to retrolental fibroplasia. Collapse of alveoli as oxygen is absorbed is, however, a more common problem associated with a high F_IO_2. It may be difficult to protect the patient from the oxygen toxicity syndrome. Intermittent exposure to lower oxygen concentrations may help but it is not usually possible. The patient treated with IPPV may be particularly at risk and high-flow oxygen through a face mask or the use of a CPAP mask should be attempted first if possible.

Bronchodilators

An obstructive component is common in patients receiving respiratory support on the ITU. A bronchodilator is therefore valuable. The first-line treatment is usually either salbutamol or ipratropium or both combined, given by nebuliser. Intravenous therapy may be required if the patient does not respond to nebulised therapy. The following pharmacological agents may be of value:

- Sympathomimetic drugs (beta agonists), e.g. adrenaline, salbutamol, isoprenaline, terbutaline, orciprenaline
- Phosphodiesterase inhibitors (increase intracellular c-AMP), e.g. aminophylline
- Steroids, e.g. hydrocortisone, prednisolone
- Drugs which stabilise mast cell membrane, e.g. disodium chromoglycate
- Anaesthetic agent with a bronchodilator effect, e.g. ketamine, isoflurane

Respiratory stimulants

Respiratory stimulants are not used often on the ITU but may be indicated when the respiratory drive is insufficient to prevent a progressively increasing P_aCO_2 (hypoxia can be treated with oxygen). They should not be used in the patient who is obviously distressed and working maximally in an attempt to maintain gaseous exchange, e.g. the patient in status asthmaticus. Doxapram has a place in the management of patients with respiratory depression due to centrally acting drugs such as the barbiturates or narcotics.

Intermittent positive pressure ventilation

When spontaneous respiratory activity is insufficient, mechanical inflation of the lungs is indicated. Humidification of respired gases will be required.

MAINTENANCE OF THE AIRWAY

Non-irritant endotracheal tubes, nasal or oral, are used:

Nasal	— advantages	Less relative movement; easy to keep mouth clean; patient can drink and eat.
	— disadvantages	Greater length; narrower bore; greater resistance; difficulty with aspiration of secretions; damage to nasal mucosa is possible.
Oral	— advantages	Easier to insert usually; aspiration of secretions is fairly easy.
	— disadvantages	Moves with swallowing or chewing; not too easy to fix securely; mouth toilet more difficult.

| Tracheostomy | — advantages | Better tolerated than an oral or nasal tube; reduced dead space; easier secretion control. |
| | — disadvantages | Surgical or invasive procedure; requires consent; haemorrhage. |

MODES OF VENTILATION

Continuous mandatory ventilation (CMV)
This is rarely used in the ITU because of its lack of flexibility and the need for a heavily sedated or paralysed patient.

Synchronised intermittent mandatory ventilation (SIMV)
This mode is common. It allows the patient to breathe between controlled breaths, is more comfortable and can be used for weaning. An unsedated patient will often tolerate SIMV. There is no evidence that SIMV accelerates weaning.

Pressure-controlled ventilation (PCV)
A relatively new technique, which is based on the old technique of pressure cycling. The ventilator delivers gas to a set maximum inspiratory pressure at a chosen rate. Tidal volume is therefore determined by lung compliance and resistance. May be an advantage in patients with ARDS but heavy sedation is usually required.

Inverse-ratio ventilation (IRV)
This basic mode may be CMV, SIMV or PCV and the I:E ratio is then adjusted such that inspiration is longer than expiration. Ratios of 2:1 or even 3:1 can be used and may improve gas exchange. Gas trapping may occur with a high PEEP.

High-frequency ventilation (HFV)
Used infrequently, HFV is advantageous in patients with a bronchopleural fistula or air leak. The risk of barotrauma is less than with conventional ventilation. Early claims of advantages over conventional ventilatory modes have not been upheld.

Positive end expiratory pressure (PEEP)
A PEEP of up to about 10 cmH$_2$O is commonly used. It increases the FRC and enhances gas exchange. Higher levels of PEEP offer no advantages and increase the risk of barotrauma.

Continuous positive airways pressure (CPAP)
This is the maintenance of up to 10 cmH$_2$O of airways pressure in a spontaneouly breathing patient. Gas exchange is enhanced and weaning promoted.

Pressure support (PS)
The application of up to 20 cmH$_2$O of PS augments inspiratory volume and promotes weaning.

MONITORING VENTILATION

A nurse-to-patient ratio of 1:1 is recommended. All modern ITU ventilators have multiple alarm systems. These should include, as a minimum, inspired oxygen, power and gas supplies, disconnection and high airway pressure. In addition, the tidal volume, rate and PEEP also commonly have alarms.

The principal aim of controlled ventilation is the maintenance of acceptable gas exchange. The final monitor of ventilation is therefore arterial blood gases and they should be measured as often as clinically indicated. As a general rule, P_aO_2 should not be allowed to fall below about 9.3 kPa or P_aCO_2 rise above about 8 kPa. These figures may need to be modified in the light of clinical circumstances. As a general rule, oxygenation is modified by both inspired concentration and minute volume while carbon dioxide removal depends on minute volume. Both are affected by PEEP, PS, I:E ratio.

ADDITIONAL CONSIDERATIONS

The patient receiving artificial ventilation will require regular physiotherapy and humidification of inspired gases (p. 182). Antibiotics may be required if there is evidence of infection. Mucolytic agents and bronchodilators may be administered by nebuliser. In patients with critical gas exchange or elevated pulmonary artery pressures, nebulised prostacyclin or inhaled nitric oxide may be used. Progressive deterioration in gas exchange may necessitate consideration of extra-corporeal gas exchange (ECMO or IVOX) for which the patient may need to be transferred to another centre. The patient, however, may be too unstable to tolerate a journey. Artificial ventilation is associated with a number of hazards which include infection, pneumothorax, barotrauma, oxygen toxicity and a reduction in cardiac output.

DISCONTINUANCE OF VENTILATION (WEANING)

Most patients can be weaned easily and quickly from the ventilator but some require weaning to be a prolonged and gradual process and indeed present a protracted problem. The patient's condition must be optimal: no heart failure, pyrexia, anaemia or abdominal splinting. Bronchospasm and secretions must be minimal. A vital capacity of at least 10 ml.kg^{-1} is thought necessary to achieve weaning; also a V_D/V_T ratio of less than 0.6 and an ability to generate at least −20 cmH$_2$O pressure on inspiration.

TECHNIQUES

1. Intermittent periods of spontaneous respiration—possible danger of hypoxia and fatigue
2. Triggering on SIMV with slowly reducing rate—commonly used
3. Mandatory minute ventilation—not in common usage—it has a theoretical advantage over SIMV, in that the minute ventilation is controlled
4. Continuous positive airway pressure (CPAP)—this may be used alone, or in conjunction with IMV and may assist weaning
5. Pressure support—reduces work of breathing and augments inspiratory volumes

SEPTICAEMIA

Patients in the ITU are more susceptible to infection than other patients. Their immune systems may be compromised, they may have a number of invasive lines in situ and resistant bacteria all around. One source of bacteria which is impossible to eradicate is the gut, and movement of bacteria across into the circulation may occur in critically ill patients. Septicaemia is, by definition, a state where micro-organisms are growing in the blood. It may not always be possible to prove this. There is progression on to the sepsis syndrome which is probably mainly due to endotoxin and other mediators released by the presence of endotoxin. Cardiac index rises and systemic vascular resistance falls. Despite (commonly) a normal or raised oxygen delivery, oxygen extraction by the tissues is impaired, leading to ischaemia. The slowly worsening peripheral ischaemia leads to steadily developing failure of vital organs and the patient usually dies of multiple oxygen failure (MOF). When more than three systems are failing for more than three days, the mortality is almost 100%.

The treatment of the sepsis syndrome is usually very dificult. Full cardiovascular and respiratory support are required. Active search should continue for sources of sepsis and, if appropriate, these should be surgically treated. The counsel of perfection is not to administer an antibiotic without proof of infection and sensitivity data. In practice this is very difficult. A number of other management regimes have been proposed and are occasionally used in some units, including selective decontamination of the gut, high doses of steroids and antioxidant therapy. The evidence that any of these are of benefit is somewhat tenuous. Anti-endotoxin antibody is available but is extremely expensive and, there is no good evidence that it is of benefit.

RENAL FAILURE

Renal failure may be defined as the inability of the kidney to excrete waste products and to maintain fluid and electrolyte balance. The serum creatinine will be raised. Urea may be raised for other reasons: dehydration, catabolism or blood in the intestine in addition to renal failure. The diagnosis of acute renal failure depends almost entirely on the changes in the biochemistry of the patient as the urine flow may be normal, high or low. In the patient with acute renal failure signs and symptoms of uraemia are often a late sign.

Patients with chronic renal failure may suddenly deteriorate and are usually admitted to hospital with uraemia. The symptoms and signs of uraemia include: lethargy, fits, thirst, vomiting, anorexia, haematemesis, air hunger, hiccup and coma. A systematic approach should be made to the differential diagnosis of acute renal failure but the uraemic patient should first be treated, and then the differential diagnosis considered (Fig. 5.4).

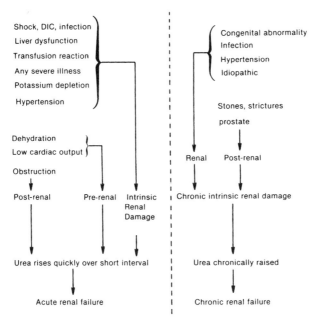

Fig 5.4   Renal failure

Investigation of acute renal failure (Fig. 5.5)

1. Discover and treat primary disorder if possible (pre-renal, renal, or post-renal).
2. Preserve veins on forearms for later dialysis.
3. Maintain strict asepsis for all invasive procedures.
4. Careful fluid balance (use a weigh-bed if necessary).
5. Maintain nutritional status (starvation accentuates uraemia).
6. Dialysis as required under the guidance of the renal physicians.
7. Correct anaemia if less than 8 g/dl.

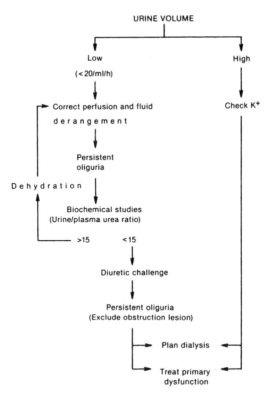

Fig 5.5 Acute renal failure

Peritoneal dialysis

Diffusion and osmosis take place across the peritoneum—a semi-permeable membrane. Small molecules move freely according to their concentration gradients. Water molecules move in accordance with the laws of osmosis. Dialysis fluids are usually dextrose solutions and are designed for specific purposes—their osmolality determines the amount of water removed, and their electrolyte concentrations the amount of electrolytes removed. Hazards of peritoneal dialysis include infection, hypovolaemia (removal of too much water), hyperglycaemia (dialysate osmolality determined mainly by its dextrose concentration), haemorrhage, diaphragmatic splinting and hypoproteinaemia. Peritoneal dialysis requires the insertion of a catheter (e.g. Tenckoff) into the peritoneal cavity. It is a technique which is underused in the intensive care unit.

Haemodialysis

Diffusion, osmosis and ultrafiltration are possible. Ultrafiltration is the result of pressurising blood in contact with the artificial semipermeable membrane so that the water is forced through into the dialysis fluid. For short-term haemodialysis an exteriorised shunt is often inserted between artery and vein, usually on the forearm or ankle, or a double-lumen cannula is inserted into a central vein. For long-term haemodialysis an arteriovenous fistula is constructed. Dialysis is tailored to suit the patient. Electrolyte correction, extraction of water and timing are all considered. Hazards include hypotension, hypovolaemia, infection, clotting of shunt and mechanical failure. In addition, the patient requires to be temporarily anticoagulated.

Haemofiltration

This is similar in nature to haemodialysis in that blood is passed one side of a semipermeable membrane and waste products and water cross. The principal differences are that a slightly different type of membrane is used, hydrostatic pressure is not used and the process is allowed to run continuously. In haemodiafiltration, a suitable dialysate is passed across the other side of the membrane. In all cases the patient requires to be anticoagulated (both heparin and prostacyclin are commonly used) and the filtrate needs to be collected and removed hourly so that replacement fluid (physiological salt solution) can be given to maintain the appropriate fluid, electrolyte and acid–base balance.

LIVER FAILURE

May be acute on a normal or chronic background or fulminant. The commonest causes of acute liver failure are viral hepatitis, drug induced or paracetamol overdose. Acute or chronic, it is usually precipitated by an insult, e.g. GI bleed, sepsis or surgery.

Clinical manifestations

Hepatomegaly, ascites and jaundice may be present. Splenomegaly is suggestive of pre-existing chronic liver disease. The cardiac output is commonly raised and the peripheral resistance is lowered. Arterio-venous shunting occurs and hypotension is frequent. Fluctuating mental changes are present, from normal consciousness to coma, and hepatic encephalopathy may be graded (Table 5.3). A false neurotransmitter may be the cause of coma and cerebral oedema or excess circulating ammonia contributing factors. Hypoxia and hypoglycaemia may be present, the latter possibly resulting from an increase in insulin levels. The mental changes are reversible but metabolic brain damage can occur, resulting in convulsions and cerebral oedema, which may not be reversible.

Table 5.3   Grading of hepatic encephalopathy

Grading	Symptoms
Grade 1	Altered mood
	Restlessness
	Decreased attention span
Grade 2	Confusion
	Lethargy
Grade 3	Deteriorating consciousness
Grade 4	Coma

Ammonia stimulates ventilation to produce respiratory alkalosis although a metabolic alkalosis is also common. Renal failure (the hepatorenal syndrome, an acute tubular necrosis) may also occur. Uraemia may be the result of the absorption of blood from the gut. There may be a coagulopathy where clotting factors are decreased and prothrombin time increased.

Management
Monitoring of ECG, BP and CVP is essential. A pulmonary artery catheter may be required. Dextrose is the safest intravenous fluid. Blood sugar should be monitored regularly because hypoglycaemia is common. Avoid absorption of toxic material from the bowel by the use of neomycin, lactulose and reducing dietary protein intake. No sedation should be prescribed, even if the patient is restless. Endotracheal intubation may be necessary to prevent aspiration, and IPPV is necessary if gas exchange is severely impaired. Electrolyte derangement, commonly hypokalaemia, may require potassium supplements and a severe metabolic alkalosis may require correction. Hypovolaemia is badly tolerated—treat adequately with careful attention to the cardiovascular parameters. Inotropic support may be required.

Some hepatologists recommend the insertion of an ICP line to aggressively treat ICP changes (see p. 84). Haemodialysis or haemofiltration may be necessary. In certain patients artificial liver support and possibly transplantation may be required. Seek the advice of a specialist centre early. H_2 receptor antagonists are needed to reduce incidence of gastric erosions. Bleeding from oesophageal varices may be controlled by using a Sengstaken–Blakemore tube. Anticipate, search for and treat infection.

ACUTE PANCREATITIS

The principal causes of acute pancreatitis are gallstones or alcohol, although there are many aetiological factors. An attack begins with acute epigastric pain, nausea and vomiting, and most attacks are self-limiting. A small number progress and require intensive care. The mortality used to be high but has dropped in recent years, probably due to more aggressive medical and surgical treatment. The patients are usually hypotensive with tachycardia, oliguria, tachypnoea and a reduced conscious level. The amylase is usually grossly elevated and there may be deranged liver function tests and hypocalcaemia. CT scan and abdominal ultrasound examination are useful to confirm the diagnosis.

Management
1. Aggressive resuscitation and invasive monitoring are required. Intravenous fluids should be given to maintain acceptable urine output and filling pressures. Blood, platelets and clotting factors will be required.
2. Intubation, controlled ventilation and increased inspired oxygen concentration.
3. Adequate analgesia (often high doses are required).
4. Nasogastric tube on free drainage.
5. Start parenteral nutrition early.
6. Surgical debridement of the diseased pancreas. The abdomen is left open and packed. The patient returns to the operating theatre every 48–72 hours for change of packs and further debridement as necessary. It may take several weeks for healing to occur.
7. Antioxidant therapy has shown promise in reducing mortality and morbidity. High doses of selenium, acetylcysteine and vitamin C are given by continuous infusion.
8. Haemofiltration or haemodiafiltration should be instituted early for renal suppport and fluid management.
9. The development of septicaemia and/or ARDS is common and should be managed accordingly.

BURNS

The commonest cause of burns in children is thermal injury (scalds) and in adults fire or hot objects, e.g. falling against a radiator. Chemical and electrical burns also occur. A high index of suspicion must be maintained for accompanying injuries, e.g. head, cervical spine or chest injuries. The burn may be secondary to a myocardial infarction, cerebrovascular incident, fit, etc. A full examination of the patient is essential.

Fluid therapy
The percentage area of burns (Wallace rule of 9s) should be calculated:

Head	—	9%
Arms	—	9% each
Legs	—	18% each
Trunk	—	18% front
		18% back
Perineum	—	1%

The areas should be graded into superficial, partial or full thickness. Burnt skin leads to a loss of water, loss of heat and bacterial colonisation. Secondary changes throughout the body include increased capillary permeability (and marked oedema formation), the release of vasoactive intermediaries, pyrexia and gross catabolism. Renal failure may develop. Fluid must be given according to a formula. The commonest is the Mount Vernon formula:

$$\text{Replacement fluid (ml)} = \frac{\text{\% burn} \times \text{body weight (kg)}}{2}$$

This volume should be given over the first 4 hours and then repeated over 4, 4, 6, 6, 12 hours. Some departments use colloid, e.g. albumin solution, gelatin or starch solution, some use crystalloid—there is no general agreement on which is best. Blood transfusions should be given as needed. The use of a central venous pressure line to guide fluid replacement is recommended.

Respiratory care
A respiratory burn must be suspected if the face, oral mucosa or nasal hairs are burnt. The larynx, trachea and main bronchi are damaged by heat, but the lesser bronchi and bronchioles are affected mainly by carbon particles or chemical irritants. Bronchospasm and pulmonary oedema are the major results of respiratory burns. The bronchospasm is unresponsive to bronchodilators, although steroids and humidification may help. Early bronchial lavage with isotonic sodium bicarbonate has been claimed to reduce morbidity and help to remove carbon particles. If marked pneumonic changes occur, the mortality rate is high. Blood gas analysis should be carried out as frequently as the clinical condition of the patient dictates and the carbon monoxide level should also be monitored.

General management
1. The haemoglobin, haematocrit, urea and electrolytes are measured as frequently as necessary. Plasma sodium concentration may be used as an indicator of the state of hydration.
2. Urinary catheterisation is required because a good urine output must be maintained to 'wash out' free Hb from the circulation and kidneys.
3. Begin feeding early—use the enteral route if possible.
4. Bacterial monitoring of burnt areas.
5. Regular chest X-rays.
6. Administer tetanus toxoid.
7. Environmental temperature and humidity should be high (32°C, 40% humidity). Heat is lost by evaporation. Heat loss can be reduced by enclosing burnt limbs in polythene bags

and by maintaining a high humidity. The calories lost by evaporation must be replaced by hyperalimentation.

8. Surgical management—early escharotomies, skin grafting and dressing with Flamazine.
9. Analgesia is required for frequent dressing changes. Entonox, ketamine or intravenous opiates are all used.
10. Anaesthesia is required for major procedures. Suxamethonium may produce a rise in potassium concentration and a cardiac arrest. It is safe for the first 48–72 hours. Repeated anaesthetics may be required and the choice of agents should reflect this possibility.

NUTRITIONAL SUPPORT OF THE ILL PATIENT

Following major trauma or surgery, muscle tissue undergoes catabolism which increases urinary nitrogen. This loss is not affected by nutrition but feeding high-energy, high-protein diets leads to a deposition of protein, partially compensating for the endogenous loss. The nitrogenous losses are maximal between the fifth and seventh days, but the degree of catabolism is less with increasing age, less in females and less if the patient has previously been in a state of undernutrition.

Enteral nutrition
Liquid feed taken enterally avoids many complications associated with the intravenous route and is cheaper. Patients incapable of swallowing or having no desire to eat or drink may be fed via a fine-bore nasogastric tube or a jejunostomy. The position of the tube should be verified by X-ray before beginning feeding. The feed may contain whole protein, peptides or free amino acids. Patients with a reduced proteolytic or absorptive capacity should be given the latter ('elemental') diets.

Diarrhoea is unlikely if the concentration or volume of the feed is gradually built up over several days. If it occurs, it may be controlled by codeine phosphate, but lactose intolerance should not be overlooked and a lactose-free feed should be instituted if necessary.

It is usual to administer the feed continuously over 24 hours via a roller pump. Some units interrupt the feeding overnight. Alternatively the patient may be fed overnight to supplement daytime intake. Prokinetic drugs may be needed, e.g. erythromycin, metoclopramide or cisapride.

Parenteral nutrition
Subclavian or internal jugular catheters tunnelled below the skin are the percutaneous venous routes of choice. The nitrogen requirements are given in the form of amino acids and the calories in the form of dextrose and lipid emulsions. The amino acid solutions available are classified in terms of their ability to deliver

nitrogen. They are complex solutions and the reasons for their composition are beyond the scope of this book. Once the desired amount of nitrogen, in g/24h, has been determined, the appropriate solution is selected. Dextrose and lipids are given either separately or the whole may be combined in large volume bags (usually 3 litres) over 24 hours.

There are two ways to determine the amount of nitrogen and dextrose that are required. The starting point can be either a calculation of nitrogen losses or an assessment of calorie requirements. The first method, although giving a precise value, involves a delay in that the results are always at least 24 h out of date, usually more. Calorie requirements can be determined from nitrogen needs and vice versa. However, the 'kcal/g nitrogen' ratio varies with the patient's clinical condition: in the non-catabolic patient the ratio may be 250:1, and in the catabolic 150:1.

An insulin infusion may be required to control blood sugar levels, and to reduce urinary losses of sugar. The infusion rate may need to be high, as insulin resistance occurs. The blood sugar requires measuring hourly and adjustments must be made to the insulin infusion rate. Sliding scales exist and the scale of choice should be designed to prevent large swings in blood glucose levels.

Water and electrolyte balance must be maintained. Attention also needs to be given to vitamins (water-soluble and lipid-soluble) and essential minerals and trace elements.

MANAGEMENT OF POISONING

Assessment
- Name of drug(s), amount taken, time taken
- Neurological status
  - Level of consciousness (ability to protect the airway)
  - Confusion/restlessness/fits
  - Psychiatric assessment
  - Thermoregulation
- Cardiovascular status
  - Blood pressure
  - Peripheral perfusion
  - Myocardial irritability
- Respiratory status
  - Ventilation
  - Safety of airway
- Hepatic function—is drug hepatotoxic?
- Renal function—is drug nephrotoxic?
- Fore-gut integrity—is drug caustic?

Supportive measures
1. Protect the airway if necessary (endotracheal tube). Intermittent positive pressure ventilation if hypoxia or hypercapnia exists.

2. Intravenous infusion. Fluids given as necessary to maintain blood volume and perfusion. A central venous line may be necessary.
3. Monitor for cardiac dysrhythmias and treat as necessary.
4. Temperature-regulating blankets may be required.
5. Control of convulsions.

Specific measures

The aim is to reduce drug effect, absorption and enhance excretion.
1. Antidotes, e.g. opiates—naloxone; iron preparations—desferrioxamine; cyanide—Kelocyanor (dicobalt edetate).
2. Gastric lavage—the aim is to remove any remaining drug from the stomach. The time elapsed between ingestion and lavage is important and may make lavage irrelevant. Assessment of airway security is important before attempting lavage.
3. Emetics may be hazardous. Oesophageal rupture may result.
4. Enhancement of excretion:
   a. Forced diuresis. Maintenance of urinary output will allow continuous elimination of the drug. This is achieved by infusion of saline and dextrose together with a diuretic. CVP control is advisable, with meticulous attention to fluid balance. Altering the pH of urine may change the ionisation of the drug present in the tubules and if the ionisation is increased reabsorption is reduced:
   • Salicylates, barbiturates—alkaline urine
   • Amphetamines, quinine, fenfluramine—acidic urine.
   b. Peritoneal dialysis may occasionally be used.
   c. Haemodialysis or haemofiltration may be beneficial.

Barbiturates

• Clinical presentation—coma; ventilatory depression; hypotension
• Management—intubation; IPPV; plasma expansion; forced diuresis. Haemodialysis may be required.

Salicylates

• Clinical presentation—reduced level of consciousness; severe acidosis; reduced prothrombin level (bleeds easily); hypokalaemia; hyponatraemia (hypernatraemia may result from attempts to raise pH with sodium bicarbonate in the presence of a very severe acidosis).
• Treatment—gastric lavage or induced vomiting; forced alkaline diuresis; increase potassium input with infusion fluids; intravenous vitamin K; hyperventilation may be required (IPPV); peritoneal dialysis if plasma salicylate concentration > 100 mg.dl^{-1}.

Paracetamol

• Clinical presentation—impaired conscious level; hepatic damage likely if plasma paracetamol > 300 mg.ml^{-1} at 4 h or > 75 mg.ml^{-1} at 12 h; prothrombin time is prolonged; hypoglycaemia; metabolic acidosis; acute renal failure.

- Treatment—measure plasma paracetamol level. Acetyl cysteine or methionine may prevent hepatic damage if given within 10–12 hours. Graphs are available of plasma paracetamol against time for treatment. If the concentration lies above the line, treatment is required. If below the line, treatment is not needed.

Phenothiazines
- Clinical presentation—drowsiness; coma; respiratory depression; hypotension.
- Treatment—vasopressors or plasma expanders may be required to combat hypotension. IPPV may be required.

Tricyclic antidepressants
- Clinical presentation—coma; respiratory depression; convulsions; cardiac dysrhythmias (tachycardia, atrial flutter, atrio- and intra-ventricular block).
- Treatment—phentolamine if hypertension occurs. Symptomatic treatment of convulsions and cardiac dysrhythmias. Monitor for cardiac dysrythmias.

Paraquat
There is progressive and lethal pulmonary fibrosis.

Treatment — Prevent further absorption (500 ml of 30% Fuller's earth and 5% magnesium)
— Haemoperfusion over activated charcoal or carbon exchange resin
— Propranolol competes with paraquat binding sites
— Forced diuresis or haemodialysis
— Lower P_aO_2 5.5 to 8 kPa. The toxic effect of paraquat is similar to that of oxygen toxicity and thus high inspired oxygen concentrations should be avoided.

Carbon monoxide
- Clinical presentation—no symptoms if < 10%; higher levels cause dyspnoea, headache, convulsions, coma, respiratory depression.
- Treatment—raise F_IO_2 to 100% or treat with hyperbaric oxygen; search for other drugs and treat accordingly; use mannitol if there are signs of raised intracranial pressure.

Organophosphorous insecticides—anticholinesterases
- Clinical presentation—pulmonary oedema, bradycardia, hypotension, nausea, vomiting, salivation, sweating, blurred vision, convulsions.
- Treatment — atropine. It may be needed repeatedly, intravenously in 2 mg boluses at 10-minute intervals, or by infusion, until symptoms are controlled.
— Pralidoxime chloride, 1–2 g i.v. (500 mg.min^{-1})
— Anticonvulsants

DIAGNOSIS OF BRAIN DEATH

Preconditions
1. The cause of the coma must be known
2. Hypothermia must be excluded
3. Electrolyte abnormalities and metabolic causes of coma must be excluded
4. Drug effects must be excluded

Criteria
- Brain function should be assessed twice by two independent doctors, one of whom must be a consultant and both must have been qualified for > 5 years
- No spontaneous motor activity
- No response to deep pain
- No cough reflex
- No pupillary response to light
- No corneal reflex
- No gag reflex
- No ocular-vestibular reflexes (caloric testing)
- No spontaneous respiration in the presence of $P_aCO_2 > 8$ kPa
- P_aO_2 should be normal or raised

The legal implications of terminating treatment vary from country to country. If the patient fulfils the above criteria (in the UK), the patient may be certified as dead and life support can be terminated. It must be remembered that the criteria also differ from country to country. Some require EEG or cerebral angiography before death can be confirmed and certified.

In every case where brain death is diagnosed and established, the possibility of organ donation should be considered. It is not possible to amplify on the procedures involved, criteria for harvesting organs or investigation required. The local transplant coordinator should be contacted for advice. Counselling and interviewing grieving relatives at this time can be traumatic and broaching the subject of organ donation may also be difficult. If in doubt, request help from any individual more experienced in these matters, e.g. consultant, colleague, nurse, chaplain.

6. Equipment

THE ANAESTHETIC MACHINE

There are many configurations of the anaesthetic machine. Fresh gas is delivered at 400 kPa (60 lb.inch^{-2} or 4 bar) from cylinders or pipelines and the flow is controlled by metering gases through flowmeters (rotameters). The gases are then passed to the patient via a vaporiser linked to either a reservoir bag, capacity 2 litre (paediatric 400 ml) in a high flow circuit, or to a circle system which may incorporate a ventilator.

The reservoir bag provides the gas volume to meet the patient's initial inspiratory rate (30 l.min^{-1}) at the anaesthetic machine flow of 6 l.min^{-1}. Anaesthetic machine outlet obstruction can cause gas pressure to rise and damage the rotameters and vaporisers unless a pressure relief valve which opens at 35 kPa is fitted between the vaporisers and the final gas outlet. Ventilators driven by anaesthetic gases usually require 20 kPa to function.

BULK GAS STORAGE

LIQUID OXYGEN

Liquid oxygen is transported, by road, in double-walled spherical containers; the outer wall is steel and the inner copper. This container, which resembles the Dewar flask, contains enough liquid oxygen to produce 100 000 ft^3 on evaporation and is used to 'top up' the smaller, but similarly designed, hospital storage tanks. The liquid oxygen is usually stored at a pressure below 1212 kPa and at a temperature maintained lower than the critical temperature of −119°C.

The critical temperature is that temperature above which an increase in pressure cannot produce liquefaction. Therefore cylinders are never completely filled with liquefied gas as a rise in temperature might result in very high pressures and cylinder rupture.

PIPELINES

Oxygen, nitrous oxide, Entonox, vacuum and compressed air can be supplied by pipeline at 400 kPa, connected to the anaesthetic and other apparatus by colour-coded flexible hoses (N_2O–blue, oxygen–white) and non-interchangeable connectors. The gases may be stored centrally in banks of large cylinders. Auditory and visual alarm devices may be used to warn of a failure in the pipe supply.

CYLINDERS

Gas storage cylinders are, for strength, manufactured from molybdenum steel. Three types of cylinder mechanical testing are used (one in every batch or one in every hundred cylinders produced is tested):

1. Tensile test. Tests are made on strips cut longitudinally from finished cylinders. The strips are tensioned until they elongate (yield).
2. Flattening, impact and bend tests. The middle half of an empty cylinder is placed between two compression blocks. The impact and bend tests stress the metal to the point of cracking.
3. Hydraulic and/or pressure test. The cylinder is enclosed in a vessel filled with water and simultaneously the pressure of water within the cylinder is increased. The change in the volume of the cylinder on applying and after removal of the internal hydraulic pressure is measured by changes in the level of water in the vessel.

IDENTIFICATION AND MARKING OF CYLINDERS

1. Cylinders are painted externally as follows:

	Valve end	*Body*
Oxygen	White	Black
Nitrous oxide	Blue	Blue
Cyclopropane	Orange	Orange
Carbon dioxide	Grey	Grey
Helium	Brown	Brown
Nitrogen	Black	Grey
O_2 and CO_2	White and grey	Black
O_2 and He	White and brown	Grey
Air	White and black	Grey
N_2O/O_2	White and blue	Blue

2. Each gas cylinder bears a label showing the name of the gas contained in the cylinder.
3. The name or chemical symbol is stencilled in paint on the shoulder of the cylinder.
4. Cylinder outlet valves have punched onto them:
   a. Name of the contained gas
   b. The tare weight
   c. The name of the manufacturer
   d. The cylinder size
   e. A series of dates indicating when the cylinder was subjected to hydraulic testing. Thus 81 ① means the first quarter of 1981. Plastic 'marker' rings, fixed between the cylinder and the outlet, are also used for this purpose.
   f. The serial number of the valve and cylinder.
5. The cylinder necks have punched onto them:
   a. The date of testing
   b. The serial number of the cylinder.

NON-INTERCHANGEABILITY

Non-interchangeable flush-type pin index valves prevent the connection of cylinders to the wrong flowmeter yokes (Fig. 6.1). These are fitted to all cylinders up to and including those with a 12 lb water capacity.

	Hole numbers for index pins	
Oxygen	2 and 5	
Oxygen and CO_2 (<7.5%)	2 and 6	
Nitrous oxide	3 and 5	
Cyclopropane	3 and 6	

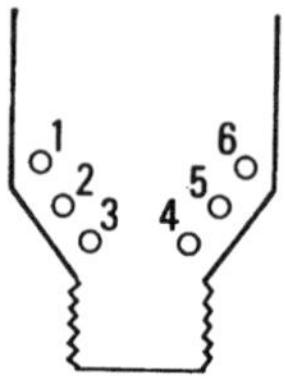

Fig 6.1   Pin index codes

'Bull-nose' valves are fitted to oxygen cylinders of a capacity exceeding 48 ft^3.The valves are designed to be non-interchangeable.

Storage pressures in kPa
Oxygen: 13.700
Nitrous oxide: 5200
Carbon dioxide: 5800
Cyclopropane: 500

PRESSURE REGULATORS/FLOW RESTRICTORS

REGULATORS

Pressure regulators control gas pressure entering the anaesthetic machine. In a low-pressure regulator the diaphragm is usually made of rubber or neoprene whereas in high-pressure regulators the diaphragms are usually metal. A two-stage regulator is used when high flow rates and large pressure reductions are required.

1. The McKesson regulator
   High-pressure reduction—metal diaphragm.
2. The Adams regulator (Fig. 6.2)
   The input may vary from 134×100 kPa (cylinder) to 402 kPa (pipeline). Because of the toggle arrangement, the pressure acting against the diaphragm moves the needle in the opposite direction, thereby occluding the high-pressure aperture.

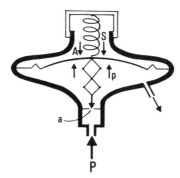

Fig 6.2 Adam's pressure reducing valve

The spring (s) and the elastic recoil of the diaphragm, distorted by the low-pressure gas, oppose the force exerted by the high-pressure gas on the needle.

Thus $Pa + s = pA$

By altering S, pressure reduction can be varied. Safety pressure release valves are often fitted on the downstream side of a regulator to offer protection to the patient in case of a regulator failure.

FLOW RESTRICTORS

Regulators are occasionally omitted when anaesthetic machines are supplied from pipelines at a pressure of 400 kPa. Sudden pressure surges are prevented at the patient end of the machine by flow restrictors fitted between the supply and the rotameters.

CHECKING BULK GAS SUPPLY AND CYLINDERS

1. Check bulk-gas warning lights
2. 'One-gas' test—this eliminates the possibility of crossed pressure hoses
   a. Confirm that the high-pressure gas hose for oxygen is connected to the correct wall outlet or large cylinder regulator and to the oxygen inlet on the anaesthetic machine
   b. Turn on the oxygen source and turn off all other gas sources
   c. After all other gases have been 'bled' from the machine, open all flow meter controls and check that oxygen only flows
3. Repeat 'one-gas' test for nitrous oxide
4. Test oxygen-supply warning device if fitted
5. Check the gas volumes in all cylinders fitted to machines. This also detects leaks and ensures that there is a key to fit each cylinder. (Note that nitrous oxide is in the liquid state—hence

vapour pressure is constant until 75% of cylinder contents have been used; also, during discharge, temperature falls and with it pressure.
6. Turn off reserve cylinders
7. Turn all wall outlets to ensure that male hose connector is firmly secured in female wall outlets

MEASUREMENT OF FLOW RATE OF GASES

The devices employed to meter the gas flow rates are:
1. The Rotameter—consists of a tapered glass tube containing a cone-shaped bobbin which has oblique notches cut in the rim to encourage its rotation. Each Rotameter is calibrated for a single gas. The scale is non-linear. Inaccuracies may occur if the tube is not vertical, is dirty, or is subjected to static electricity.
2. Ball-float meters—these also consist of a tapered tube which may be positioned vertically or at a slope. The Quantiflex gas mixer not only incorporates such a metering device but also enables the oxygen concentration to be preset.
3. The Heidbrink meter—the tube is tapered. The flow determines the position of a metal rod.

Gas flow at low flow rates is laminar and flow rate depends on viscosity (flow through a tube). At high flow rates the bobbin moves up the tube, flow is turbulent and the space between it and the tube is effectively an orifice. Gas density is the predominant factor. Turbulent flow is non-linear.

VAPORISERS

Most vaporisers offer high resistance to gas flow; the pressure within them is higher than the outside pressure (plenum vaporiser).

NON-TEMPERATURE-COMPENSATED

A fall in liquid temperature reduces vapour formation.
1. The 'Boyle' bottle (glass)
2. The Goldman vaporiser—output limited by flow rate and agent temperature
3. Copper kettle
4. The Dräger 'Vapor'
5. Bryce-Smith induction unit

TEMPERATURE-COMPENSATED

1. Hot water bath
2. Adjust gas flow through vaporiser—bimetallic strip
3. Continuous flow
   a. TEC series

b. Engstrom Elsa
c. Dräger Vapor
d. The Penlon
e. Siemens 950
4. Draw-over vaporisers
   a. PAC series
   b. Afya Dräger
   c. Oxford Miniature Vaporiser (OMV)
   d. Epstein/MacIntosh/Oxford (EMO)

VIC (VAPORISER INSIDE CIRCLE)

The patient breathes spontaneously through a vaporiser in the circle circuit so the resistance to gas flow should be low. Furthermore, as the breathed gases pass through the vaporiser several times during inspiration and expiration the inspired concentration will be higher than that set on the dial and therefore its efficiency in terms of the concentration that it can deliver should also be low. Spontaneous breathing limits anaesthetic inhalation. A high dose of anaesthetic during spontaneous breathing leads to respiratory depression. This reduces the amount of gas passed through the vaporiser and hence the inspired concentration. A VIC system should not be used in the absence of agent monitoring.

VOC (VAPORISER OUTSIDE CIRCLE)

With the vaporiser outside the circle there is no need for a low resistance to gas flow. The inspired concentration of vapour is lower than that set on the dial because the expired gases, of lower vapour concentration, dilute the vapour in the fresh gas. Intermittent positive pressure ventilation is not contraindicated.

BREATHING SYSTEMS

Breathing tubes are made of non-compliant corrugated plastic with a volume between 400 and 450 ml per metre. The corrugations prevent kinking.

WITHOUT CARBON DIOXIDE ABSORPTION

Mapleson, in 1954, classified the existing breathing systems into five groups, A–E (Fig. 6.3), depending on their re-breathing characteristics (see Table 6.1). The flow of fresh gas in each required to prevent CO_2 re-breathing has been measured.

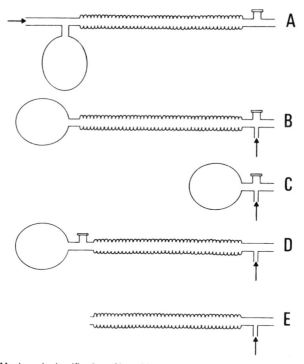

Fig 6.3 Mapleson's classification of breathing systems

Table 6.1 Mapleson-type fresh gas flow to prevent re-breathing of CO_2

		Spontaneous ventilation	Controlled ventilation
A.	Magill, Lack[*1]	0.75 VE	VA depends on mode of operation[+]
B.		2.0 VE	> 8 l.min⁻¹
C.	Water's system	2.0–3.0 VE	> 8 l.min⁻¹
D.	Bain[*2]	1.5–2.0 VE	70ml.min⁻¹.kg⁻¹
E.	Ayres T-piece/Bain[*3]	1.5–2.0 VE	$(1 + (E/I) \times V$ depends on $I{:}E$ ratio)[+]

[+] If the inspiratory time is 0.5 s and the expiratory time is 1.0 s, then the $I{:}E$ ratio would be 1:2 and the expression $I + (E/I) = 1 + 2/1 = 3$
V = fresh gas flow
*Coaxial system   1. Reservoir bag on inspiratory side
                          2. Reservoir bag on expiratory side with expiratory valve
                          3. Open ended reservoir bag on expiratory side

[+] Ventilation with the Mapleson A circuit can be achieved by:
                          1. Partially closing the expiratory relief valve and allowing a leak during the inspiratory phase

2. Completely closing the expiratory relief valve during the inspiratory phase—Carden/M.I.E. ventilator
3. Using an injector positioned between the catheter mount and the breathing system—this entrains gas from the system during inspiration and thus the flow pattern is similar to that during spontaneous ventilation

Fresh gas delivery tubing may be of narrow bore, hence high resistance, but all breathing hose must be of low resistance. In the Bain system gas is delivered through the central tube; in the Lack, it is via the outer circumferential space, the expiratory gas passing through the inner tube. Because of the flow characteristics of the Mapleson A both the inner and outer conduits of the Lack system must be of low resistance.

WITH CARBON DIOXIDE ABSORPTION

Soda lime 90% $Ca(OH)_2$. 5% NaOH, 1% KOH is used to remove carbon dioxide from the gas mixture in the breathing system.
    Silicates are included to prevent powdering and moisture present encourages the chemical reaction.
$$CO_2 + 2NaOH \rightarrow H_2O + Na_2CO_3 + heat$$
$$Na_2CO_3 + Ca(OH)_2 \rightarrow 2NaOH + CaCO_3 + heat$$
4–8 mesh granules are used to minimise the resistance to breathing and also provide an appropriate surface area for absorption. Resistance should be less than 2–3 cmH_2O at normal tidal flows.

To-and-fro system (Water's)
Advantage: Compactness
Disadvantages: 1. Absorber near patient's head—unwieldy
                        2. Apparatus dead space is high (200 ml)
                        3. Horizontal position of canister leads to channelling of gas through soda lime
                        4. Danger of inhalation of soda lime dust
                        5. If V_T < volume of soda lime canister the proximal granules become exhausted and the dead space rises

Circle systems
These systems may be semi-closed or, increasingly, totally closed. It is usual for the vaporiser to be outside the circle in the semi-closed system; however, the volatile liquid anaesthetic may be injected directly into the circuit.
    The lower the fresh gas flow the more likely are large variations from the expected gas concentrations in the circle; therefore oxygen concentration must be monitored in the inspired gas. These variations occur because of different rates of uptake of the gases in the mixture.

When the circle system is used for paediatric anaesthesia the gas may be circulated through the circuit by a fan, e.g. a Revell circulator, to ensure removal of carbon dioxide.

When using a totally closed system, anaesthetic vapour is lost. It is therefore possible to predict very accurately the amount of volatile agent required for a known time.

The advantages of the low-flow circle system are economy, humidification and stability of inhaled gas concentration once the initial equilibration phase is over. A disadvantage is that intubation is mandatory when using very low flows—to ensure a safe gas seal. The carbon dioxide absorber is held in a vertical position to reduce the likelihood of channelling of gas through the granules.

The pressure at which the relief valve operates to protect the Rotameters and vaporisers (35 kPa) is too high to protect the patient's airway from barotrauma, and therefore another valve must be incorporated in the breathing system to protect the patient in the event of obstruction to the gas outflow. This pressure-limiting valve should be set at 4–6 kPa (40–60 cmH$_2$O).

SCAVENGING

Low concentrations of anaesthetic agents in the environment are considered unacceptable; it is therefore considered desirable to exhaust all waste anaesthetic gases away from working areas.

There is some evidence that the effects of chronic exposure to anaesthetic agents are:
1. Obstetric:
   a. Increased risk of miscarriage
   b. Premature delivery
2. Headache and fatigue (theatre staff)
3. Increased incidence of malignancy in lymphoid tissue

As a gas leaves the breathing system it is ducted away, either passively or actively. Passive systems have the advantage of simplicity but exhausting the gases to the outside of buildings is not without difficulty, e.g. wind direction and other causes of obstruction, even birds' nests. Active systems are complex and require high flows (up to 130 l.min^{-1}) and negative pressures which are only slightly less than those in the breathing system. Excessive negative pressure may cause the reservoir bag to empty, making low-flow circuits impracticable. The requirement for high-flow scavenging may be reduced by using a reservoir bag in the system—to take the dumped gas during expiration and thereby even out fluctuations during the breathing cycle.

Obstruction to the scavenging tubing prevents the exhaust of the waste gases and may lead to an excessively high pressure in the airway. This can be prevented by having a safety discharge valve in the scavenging system close to the patient, opening at 0.5–1.0 kPa.

The removal of volatile agents by passing exhausted gas through activated charcoal is an alternative method. Nitrous oxide is not removed. The life of a single charcoal canister depends on the concentration of vapours passing through it and is generally about 3–6 hours. Some canisters can be recycled by passing them through an autoclave—this removes the vapour, reactivating the charcoal and exhausting the wasted gas. Exhaustion of a charcoal canister can be determined by weight.

The vacuum pumps used to extract the gases must be resistant to the effects of the vapours.

VENTILATORS

Ventilators are machines designed to deliver, by lung inflation and deflation, a mixture of gases to patients in such a way that oxygen uptake and carbon dioxide elimination are maintained. Hunter (1961), Mushin et al (1969) and Grogono (1972) have each attempted to classify ventilators.

Hunter's classification was based on either a preset tidal volume or airway pressure, Mushin's approach depended on the constancy of the flow or pressure and the method of cycling, and Grogono based his classification on whether the machine's function was independent of the patient's changing respiratory rate.

Constant-flow ventilators produce linear changes in the airway pressure, i.e. the lung volume rises linearly because of the constant flow and therefore the airway pressure will also rise linearly, assuming constant compliance if time or volume cycled. No tidal volume compensation for leaks.

Constant-pressure ventilators produce exponential changes in lung volume and flow. Compensation for leaks occurs within limits. Volume or time cycled.

Minute volume dividers, at a set rate, will produce a given airway pressure. This is because rate determines tidal volume, and tidal volume/compliance equals pressure.

A ventilator ought to be able to maintain a patient's minute ventilation even if there is an obstruction or a leak. When a change in one ventilatory parameter is made, the others should remain constant, e.g. a change in tidal volume should not produce a change in respiratory rate. Ventilators should be reliable, stable, flexible and simple to operate. Monitoring and warning devices should be available and the respiratory circuits should be removable for sterilising. Compression of gases within the machine and respiratory hoses can account for 20% of the tidal volume.

Ventilators for paediatric use should have a tidal volume in the range 10–150 ml, with rates of 30–120 min^{-1}.

There are special ventilator machines for use with neonates; however, adult machines can be adapted to manage the larger child, as follows:

1. A resistance may be inserted in parallel with the child. Some gas passes to the child and some through the resistance. This system acts as a pressure generator.
2. A compliance, e.g. a distensible bag, may be inserted in parallel. The disadvantage of this is that if the child's compliance falls then a greater volume will pass into the bag and the child's tidal volume will fall.
3. A bag or bellows in a bottle is a better arrangement—the fresh gas flow is completely separate from the adult respiratory circuit and determines the minute ventilation. The adult ventilator simply squeezes the bag or bellows within the bottle.

Trigger, intermittent mandatory ventilation (IMV) and mandatory minute ventilation (MMV) are three techniques which assist the weaning of patients off ventilators.

A trigger is effective only if the response time of the ventilator to the patient's inspiratory effort is brief enough to deliver the set tidal volume during the inspiratory effort, and not during the expiratory phase that follows. The pressure required to trigger the ventilator can be increased as the patient's respiratory ability improves.

IMV is a technique during which the mechanical tidal volume and frequency of ventilation are preset, the patient being free to breathe spontaneously between the mandatory inflations. However, the patient may have difficulty in synchronising with the ventilator when the controlled breaths are too infrequent.

MMV is a similar system; however, the total minute ventilation is determined by the fresh gas flow. Gas which the patient does not breathe spontaneously is diverted to a minute volume divider and is used to ventilate the patient mechanically. This system ensures a fixed minute volume, thereby reducing the likelihood of carbon dioxide retention or hypoxia.

HUMIDIFIERS

The water content of inspired gas should approach 44 mg.l^{-1} 100% relative humidity at 37°C.

1. Rebreathing systems—To and fro | 40–100% saturation
   Circle | 40–60% saturation
2. Swedish 'nose'—Heat and moisture exchanger | 40–90% saturation
3. Water bath humidifiers—100% saturation. When bubbling gas through, or over, heated water it becomes 100% saturated at the water temperature. As the gas passes towards the patient it cools and water condenses. However, 100% humidity is still maintained, though the amount of water is reduced. The temperature of the gas entering the patient should be monitored.

4. Mechanical nebulisation—100% saturation. Baffles are used to break up droplets, and 80% of the droplets inhaled are sized between 2 and 4 μm. These are deposited mainly in the upper airways.
5. Ultrasonic nebulisation—more than 150% saturation possible. A crystal vibrating at a frequency of about 3 MHz nebulises droplets of water; 70% of these particles will be between 0.8 and 1 μm. Overhydration is possible, increases in airway resistance have been described, and cross-infection by contamination of the droplet aerosol has been demonstrated.

Water vapour is the ideal mode of humidication (no droplets means no cross-infection), but when droplet aerosols are used the optimal size of droplet is about 3–8 μm.

FILTERS

GAS

Filters are used in high-pressure gas lines to protect against dirt, the ventilator control circuits particularly those which are under fluidic control; other filters are found on some ventilator air entrainment inlets.

The use of bacterial gas filters within the breathing circuit is now common. Their use reduces, or avoids, the necessity for ventilator sterilisation and protects the patient from airborne cross-infection. Waterlogging of the filter increases airway resistance and facilitates the passage of bacteria through the filter. This problem has now been overcome by siliconising the filter element, a water-repellant material. Filters should be new (disposable) or autoclaved for each patient.

LIQUID

Filters may be used to prevent the entry into the circulation of a variety of small particles found in intravenous infusions and drugs; these include metal, glass, fibres, moulds, and even diatoms and insects. The pore size used is 2 μm and thus acts also as a bacterial filter. Flow rates through the filter are low and some debris can be dislodged from the filter itself. Filters are not used routinely during intravenous infusions but are generally used for the administration of epidural local anaesthetics.

BLOOD FILTERS

Aggregates in blood can be large—up to 160 μm.
The filtration of particles down to 40 μm in size removes these aggregates while allowing the normal cellular material to pass. Some filters have a pore size of 20 μm.

There are two types—screen filters and depth filters; the former are of large surface area (area being increased by multiple folds in a single layer of screen) but suffer the disadvantage of pore occlusion; however, at high flows aggregates are prevented from passing. The depth filters remove aggregates by adsorbing them on tangled fibre meshes; they tend to clog less but at high flow particles may be dislodged.

The case for the use of blood filters has not been proved, except possibly when transfusions in excess of 4 units of blood are given.

ENDOTRACHEAL TUBES

There are many designs of endotracheal tubes. The general considerations determining their construction follow.

MATERIAL

Red rubber   — not normally disposable
                 — relatively irritant, and not ideal for prolonged intubation
                 — firm/curvature predetermined
                 — may transmit infection
Plastic (PVC) — disposable
                 — non-irritant (implantation-tested)
                 — moulds to body contours at 37°C

CUFFS

Red rubber cuffs are firm and rounded so that a seal between the endotracheal tube and the trachea exists over a small area. The mucosa is likely to be damaged, not only because of the chemical irritants but also because of compression, and hence hypoxia, of the mucosa (Fig. 6.4).

PVC tubes have cuffs of varying shapes. The shape of the cuff can be more cylindrical, thus, by increasing the area of seal, there is a reduction in the pressure necessary in the cuff.

The seal between tracheal mucosa and endotracheal tube is required to prevent the escape of gas (during IPPV) and also to prevent the aspiration of saliva or gastric contents into the tracheobronchial tree.

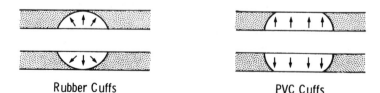

       Rubber Cuffs   PVC Cuffs

Fig 6.4   Endotracheal cuff characteristics

With low-pressure cuffs the factors that determine whether a leak will occur are:
1. The pressure in the cuff
2. The length of the cuff
3. The cohesive force between the cuff material and the mucosa, depending on surface tension
4. The duration of the inspiratory phase (the elevated pressure); the longer the pressure is applied more of the cuff will be 'stripped' away from the mucosa and the greater is the likelihood of a leak

Leakage of fluid from above the vocal cords past the cuff into the trachea depends on the head of pressure involved, and also on any movement of any fluid between the cuff and the tracheal wall in capillary-like channels.

SIZE

The outside diameter of the tube determines the smallest lumen into which it can be passed; the inside of the diameter together with the length affects air-flow resistance and hence the work of breathing. (Fig. 6.5) Resistance is measured as the pressure drop in centimetres of water along the tube for a given flow of gas; standard measurements are made at a flow of 40 $l.min^{-1}$.

It can be seen from Figure 6.5 that, for tubes with an inside diameter of greater than 7 mm, small increases in the inside diameter confer little advantage in terms of flow as r^4, although large, increases at a declining rate.

Age/4 + 4.5 is the accepted formula for determining the size (mm) of the endotracheal tube, for a child.

The length of the tube for a child is determined by:

Age/2 + 12 cm (oral)

Age/2 + 15 cm (nasal)

For infants, the largest endotracheal tube that will fit the cricoid ring, the narrowest part of the child's airway, should be passed. In tubes of small diameter, as required for infants, there is a relatively marked change in the resistance to air flow during breathing for a small difference in tube diameter. Below the age of 10 it is often considered unnecessary to use cuffed tubes; this reduces subglottic damage and enables the use of a tube of larger internal diameter. The tube should not be a tight fit.

Gas flow in endotracheal tubes with a smooth and regular inner surface is laminar at flow rates less than the critical velocity. A small tube which is contaminated with debris will induce turbulent flow. Angled connectors also produce turbulence.

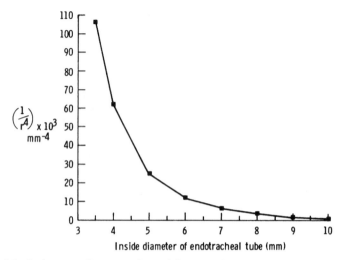

Fig 6.5　Resistance to flow versus internal diameter of endotracheal tubes

There are many different tubes; the common paediatric ones are:
1. Magill flexometallic
2. Cole
3. Plain Magill
4. Portex
5. Oxford
6. Jackson Rees

There are many specialised tubes used in adults:
1. Red rubber reinforced—styllete introducer required
2. PVC reinforced
3. Pollard and Coplans—for laryngeal microsurgery
4. Montando—for laryngectomy
5. Oxford
6. Carden—for intra-tracheal jet ventilation
7. Endobronchial/double—lumen tubes (see Table 6.2)
8. Oesophageal obturator—for emergency resuscitation
9. Rae tube—north and south facing

Table 6.2 Methods available for producing bronchial blockade
Right lung to be collapsed

Single-lumen tube	Double-lumen tube	Bronchus blocker
Machray modification[*1]	Carlen's tube	Vernon Thompson[$3] blocker right main bronchus + endotracheal tube
Magill endobronchial tube in left main bronchus		
Magill endobronchial[*1] tube in the left main bronchus	Bryce-Smith/Salt[+2] tube into right main bronchus	Magill bronchus[$3] occluder + endotracheal tube
MacIntosh–Leatherdale left endotracheal tube	Bryce-Smith tube into left main bronchus	
Brompton–Pallister left sided with one cuff on tracheal tube and two on broncheal	Left-sided Robertshaw tube	
	White right-sided[+2] (carinal hook)	

Left lung to be collapsed

Single-lumen tube	Double-lumen tube	Bronchus blocker
	Carlen's tube[+2]	Vernon Thompson[$3] blocker left main bronchus + endotracheal tube
Magill right tube[*1] with wire coil	Bryce-Smith/Salt tube into right main bronchus allows ventilation of right upper lobe	Magill bronchus occluder + endotracheal tube
MacIntosh–Leatherdale into left bronchus. Blocker and combined endotracheal tube	Bryce-Smith tube[+2] left main bronchus	
Gordon–Green right-sided tube (allows ventilation right upper lobe	Right-sided Robertshaw tube	
	White right-sided permits ventilation right upper lobe (carinal hook)	

[1*] Must be introduced over bronchoscope
[2+] Although can be used for this purpose—best avoided for pneumonectomy
[$3] Must be introduced through bronchoscope
For right upper lobectomy:
1. Magill bronchus occluder plus endotracheal tube
2. Vellacott right-sided tube ⎫ allowing ventilation of right, middle and lower
3. Green right-sided tube ⎭ lobes and left lung

Reproduced with permission of the authors and publishers, from Thornton J A, Levy C J Techniques of Anaesthesia. Chapman & Hall, London.

LARYNGOSCOPES

There are many designs for use depending on requirement:

1. NEONATAL—STRAIGHT BLADE

The epiglottis is relatively large and floppy; a straight blade is necessary to flatten and hold the epiglottis forward to allow the cords to be visualised.

2. INFANT—STRAIGHT OR CURVED BLADE

The tongue of the infant is large in relation to the buccal cavity and blade design is aimed at keeping it out of the way. Blades which are almost tubular are used in infants with tissue flaps associated with palatal defects. The most commonly used paediatric laryngoscopes are the Anderson–Magill and the Robertshaw.

3. ADULT—STRAIGHT OR CURVED BLADE

The primary aim is deflection of the tongue from the line of vision of the vocal cords; however, a variety of other problems have been overcome.
a. A laryngoscope with an obtuse angle between the handle and the blade—to facilitate insertion into the mouths of patients with difficult access, e.g. in an iron lung, in severe fixed flexion or in a halo splint for stabilisation of the cervical spine.
b. A 'left–handed blade'—for use in patients where the right side of the mouth is invaded by tumour, or access is otherwise compromised.
c. The addition of a prism to the blade allows the vocal cords to be visualised when they are not in direct line of sight.
d. McCoy Laryngoscope. Resembles a conventional laryngoscope, but the distal part of the blade is hinged and can be tilted up or down by a lever on the handle. Allows the larynx to be 'lifted' to improve vision in case of difficulty.

4. LARYNGEAL MASK AIRWAY (LMA)

A revolution in airway control. The LMA is inserted into the mouth and advanced until it comes to lie against the posterior pharyngeal wall opposite the larynx. The large cuff is then inflated and this creates a seal around the laryngeal opening. The seal of airway to trachea is not so reliable as when using an endotracheal tube and a number of studies have shown some leakage past the LMA which could potentially enter the trachea. Some doubts have been expressed as to the suitability of the LMA for use during controlled ventilation and for surgery within the mouth and pharynx, e.g., tonsillectomy. Nevertheless, it has been used widely for these situations. Great care must be taken to ensure that airway inflation pressures remain low if using an LMA for controlled ventilation.

5. FIBREOPTIC LARYNGOSCOPE

A thin flexible fibreoptic device that will pass through a tracheal tube. The fibrescope is passed through the nose or mouth (the nose is usually easier) and advanced under direct vision until it lies within the trachea. The tracheal tube, which has been previously slid onto the fibrescope is then advanced using the fibrescope as a guide. The fibrescope is then withdrawn. The use of the fibreoptic laryngoscope requires previous training. It is the safest technique for securing the airway in case of anticipated difficult intubation and may be performed with the patient awake following local analgesia to the airway.

Index